**This book is to be returned on or before
the last date stamped below.**

D1583521

A Colour Atlas of
Nutritional Disorders

Donald S. McLaren

MD, Ph.D, MRCP(Edin.), DTM&H
Reader in Clinical Nutrition,
Department of Medicine,
Royal Infirmary, Edinburgh.

Formerly Professor of Clinical Nutrition,
School of Medicine,
American University of Beirut, Lebanon.

Wolfe Medical Publications Ltd

Copyright © D.S. McLaren 1981

Published by Wolfe Medical Publications Ltd, 1981

Printed by Royal Smeets-Weert, Netherlands

ISBN 0 7234 0757 6

This book is one of the titles in the series of
Wolfe Medical Atlases, a series which brings
together probably the world's largest systematic
published collection of diagnostic colour
photographs.
For a full list of Atlases in the series, plus
forthcoming titles and details of our surgical,
dental and veterinary Atlases, please write to
Wolfe Medical Publications Ltd, 3 Conway Street,
London W1P 6HE

Contents

Acknowledgements

The author and publishers would like to thank the following for provision of the figures listed below:

1 Professor Dr W. Sandritter. 2 & 3 Dr S.P. Allison. 8 Professor J.D.L. Hansen. 9 Professor D. Morley. 11 Dr I. Maddocks. 12 Professor D. Morley. 17 Dr H.A.P.C. Oomen. 20–22 Dr F. Mönckeberg B. 23–26 Dr H. Grossman. 27 Professor R. Hendricksen. 28–30 Dr H.A.P.C. Oomen. 43 & 44 Dr J.J.M. Sauter. 45–48 Dr R.R. Pfister. 56–58, 68 & 69 Dr J.J.M. Sauter. 70 Dr A. Sommer. 71 Dr H.H. Sandstead. 74 Dr M.D. Muenter. 75 & 76 Dr H. Grossman. 77–79 Dr I.A. Abrahamson, Snr. 80 Dr A. Bryceson. 81 Professor A.J. Radford. 82 & 83 Dr C.S. Treip. 92, 93, 98 & 100 Dr H.H. Sandstead. 105–107 Dr M.K. Horwitt. 111 & 112 Dr R.W. Vilter. 113 Dr A.C. Parker. 114 Dr W.R. Tyldesley. 115 & 116 Dr A.C. Parker. 117 Professor A.V. Hoffbrand. 118 Dr W.R. Tyldesley. 119 Dr M. Zatouroff. 120 & 121 Dr E.J. Watson-Williams. 122 Dr C.S. Treip. 123 Mr M.A. Bedford. 124–127 Dr C.E. Butterworth, Jnr. 128 & 129 Dr L.S. Taitz. 130 Dr C.W. Woodruff. 131 Dr H.E. Sandstead. 132 & 133 Dr R.W. Vilter. 134 & 135 Dr C.W. Woodruff. 136 Dr R.W. Vilter. 137 Dr H.H. Sandstead. 138 Dr H.M. Gilmour. 139 & 140 Dr R.W. Vilter. 141 Dr C.W. Woodruff. 142 Dr R.W. Vilter. 143 Professors W. Peters and H.M. Gilles. 144 Professor J.M. Farquhar. 146 & 147 Dr H.M. Gilmour. 149–151 Professor J.M. Farquhar. 152 Professor A. Prader. 153 Dr M. Gebre-Medhin. 154 & 155 Dr C. Thomas, Jnr. 156 Dame Sheila Sherlock. 157–160 Professor J.O. Forfar. 161 & 162 Dr C.S. Foster. 163 & 164 Dr M. Dynski-Klein. 165 & 166 Dr M.C. Riella. 167 & 168 Dr A.C. Parker. 169 Dr A.J. Salsbury. 170 Dr M. Zatouroff. 171 & 172 Dr H. Grossman. 173–185 Dr L-G Larrson. 186 Dr M. Zatouroff. 187 Dr A.C. Parker. 188 & 189 Dr H.M. Gilmour. 190 Dr M. Zatouroff. 191 Dr H.M. Gilmour. 195 Dr R. Hall. 196 Dr M. Dynski-Klein. 197 Dr J.T. Dunn. 198 & 199 Dr H.M. Gilmour. 201 Mr L.W. Kay. 206 Dr M. Dynski-Klein. 207, 209 Dr L. Finberg. 210 & 211 Dr V. Parsons. 213 & 214 Dr C.S. Treip. 215 Dame Sheila Sherlock. 216–218 Dr J.M. Walshe. 219 Dr D.M. Danks. 220 & 221 Dr A. Kennedy. 222–225 Dr J.F. Sullivan. 226 Dr M. Dynski-Klein. 227 & 228 Dr M. Zatouroff. 229–231 Dr M. Dynski-Klein. 232 Professor Dr W. Sandritter. 233 & 234 Dr M. Zatouroff. 235 Mr M.A. Bedford. 236 Dr M. Zatouroff. 237 Mr M.A. Bedford. 238–240 Dr H.M. Gilmour. 241–243 Dr S.M. Podos. 244 Dr R. Hall. 245 Mr Ching. 246 & 247 Dr R.R. Howell. 248 Dr S.M. Podos. 249 Professor K. Weinbren. 250 Professor J.M. Farquhar. 251 Dr von G.-W. Schmidt. 253 Dr R.P. Burns. 254 Dr H. Ghadimi. 255 & 256 Dr S.H. Mudd. 257 Dr S.M. Podos. 258 Dr K. Takki. 259 Dr H.M. Gilmour. 260 Dr J.B. Wyngaarden. 261 & 262 Dr H.M. Gilmour. 263 Dr A. Ferguson. 264–266 Dr H.M. Gilmour. 267 & 268 Dr K.L. Jones. 269 Professor B. Leiber. 270 Dr D.B. Jelliffe. 271 Crown copyright © Ministry of Agriculture, Fisheries and Food. 273 Crown copyright © Tropical Products Institute. 274 Dame Sheila Sherlock. 275 Dr D.O. Gibbons. 276 & 277 Dr H.M. Gilmour. 278 Dr T. Philp. 279 Professor M.S.R. Hutt. 282 & 283 Professor C.M. Anderson. 284 Professors W. Peters and H.M. Gilles. 287 Dr H.M. Gilmour. 288 Dr T. Philp.

Preface

Although it cannot be stated categorically that all of the essential nutrients for man have been identified it is very unlikely that any of major significance to health remain to be added to the present number of about 50. The latest vitamin, vitamin B₁₂, was discovered more than 30 years ago. During that time many more trace elements have been shown to be essential for animals, and those now number 11 with 4 more of doubtful status. Most of these have been shown, or are suspected, to be essential for man and as food faddism spreads and seriously ill patients are increasingly fed parenterally with specially prepared nutrient mixtures instances of deficiency states have come to the fore. The growth of food processing with risks from contamination have increased the possibility of toxicity from some elements, as well as from other substances in food.

Despite our greatly increased understanding of the nature and extent of malnutrition problems in developing countries, there is little evidence that they are anywhere being brought under control. On the contrary, with the ever increasing world population, especially marked in developing countries, it is clear that more people are suffering from malnutrition today than ever before. The methodology of nutritional assessment has become more sensitive in recent years, particularly with the development of many biochemical tests, but these require sophisticated laboratories and trained personnel, are costly and the results are often difficult to interpret. As in the past, so in the forseeable future, detailed clinical examination for physical signs must be the most practical means of assessing nutritional status of individuals and communities, and of drawing attention to the occurrence and nature of specific nutritional deficiency states.

On the other hand it is only in recent years that recognition has been given to the important role that diet plays in most of the major causes of morbidity and mortality in technologically advanced societies. Although most of these conditions are not directly attributable to an imbalanced diet this does play a part in the aetiology of some and in others dietary measures are an important part of management. It is in these societies also, where advances in diagnosis have made possible the precise identification of the nature of many metabolic derangements, that many more conditions that were previously fatal or untreatable can now be controlled with special diets. Here too the toxic effects of excessive use of vitamins and some trace elements have to be guarded against. Furthermore, it must not be assumed that classical deficiency diseases like rickets, beriberi, scurvy and xerophthalmia need no longer concern the physician practising among over-fed rather than under-fed populations. These and other deficiency states may occur in the presence of an adequate dietary intake from impairment of the utilization of a nutrient at some stage in the body.

It should also be observed that Nutrition is not only no respecter of persons, but it is also no respecter of systems, organs or tissues. None is exempt from the harmful results of the tipping of the dietary balance beyond the limits of normal that are so difficult to define, or from a failure in utilization even when those limits are not transgressed.

One final comment may be made. The role of nutrients in the large majority of disorders dealt with in this book is clearly understood and the therapeutic and dietary means to cure or control them are available. That they together account for a high proportion of all illness throughout the world is at least in part due to failure in recognition. It is to be hoped that this atlas, the most comprehensive on the subject as far as it is known, will make a contribution towards remedying the situation.

Introduction: Definitions and Concepts

In the simplest terms *Nutrition* may be defined as *the process by which the organism utilizes food.* This process is a complicated one involving digestion, absorption, transport, storage, metabolism and elimination of the many nutrients that are to be found in the very varied diets which we call our food. All of this has as its purpose the *maintenance of life, growth, reproduction and normal functioning of organs and production of energy.*

Nutriture, or *nutritional status*, is the state of the body produced by the process and is determined by the balance between the supply of nutrients on the one hand and the expenditure by the organism on the other.

It is important to recognise that *food* and *nutrients* are not synonymous. There are many cultural, psychological and analeptic aspects to eating that are not directly concerned with the consumption of nutrients. These have to be taken into account when attempts are made to ensure an adequate intake of nutrients, especially when appetite is poor and when certain foodstuffs have to be restricted in the management of disease. Besides nutrients food may contain other substances which may have either a harmful or a beneficial effect when eaten. Food toxins are an example of the former and indigestible fibre of the latter. In certain diseases some normal food constituents are not normally metabolized and tissue damage results. Examples are gluten in coeliac disease and phenylalanine in phenylketonuria. All of these aspects are clearly related to diet and nutrition and consequently receive attention in this book.

In relation to epidemiology the concept of an Agent-Host-Environment interaction system has been developed. It is helpful to extend this to Nutrition. The Agent of Nutrition is clearly Nutriment or the Nutrients interacting with the Host; Man in this case. That part of the Environment concerned in Nutrition is the part of it we ingest, namely Food.

It is convenient to divide the nutrients into two categories, *micro-* and *macro-nutrients*. Micronutrients include vitamins and some elements. *Vitamins* are *chemical compounds occurring naturally in food and essential in small amounts for the health of the organism.* They can be divided into fat-soluble (A, D, E and K), and water-soluble vitamins (including thiamin, riboflavin, niacin, pyridoxine, folic acid and vitamin B_{12}

of the B group and vitamin C). The former tend to be stored in the body and some of their functions are not clearly understood. Except for vitamin B_{12}, water-soluble vitamins are little stored and they usually function as coenzymes.

Many *elements* are present in food and find their way into the body. Some, like calcium, phosphorus, potassium, sulphur, sodium, chlorine and magnesium, are essential for health and occur in the body in a concentration of more than 0.005%. Others, like iron, iodine, copper, zinc, manganese, cobalt, molybdenum, selenium, chromium, nickel, tin, silicon, fluorine and vanadium, are also essential but occur in smaller concentration (less than 0.005%) and are called *trace elements*. Other elements are suspected of being essential but final proof is lacking (e.g. barium, strontium). Finally elements for which no metabolic role has so far been demonstrated are absorbed occasionally (e.g. gold, silver, aluminium).

The macro-nutrients are the old 'proximate principles' (in the sense that they were the first arrived at in the process of analysis) and include carbohydrates, fats and proteins.

Micro- and macro-nutrients differ in a number of ways (see Table 1). Among the products of digestion of each of the classes of macro-nutrients, proteins, fats and carbohydrates, there is a special group segregated by essentiality and dietary requirement. These products are amino acids, fatty acids and glycerol, glucose and other monosaccharides.

Several amino acids (depending on the animal species) are called essential or indispensable as they either cannot be made at all or only in inadequate amounts by the body. For man these are lysine, tryptophan, methionine, phenylalanine, threonine, leucine, isoleucine, valine and histidine. For all but threonine and lysine the provision of the carbon skeletons is enough; there is no protein requirement as such. The requirement is for certain essential amino acids and a certain amount of non-essential nitrogen. Among fats certain polyunsaturated fatty acids are essential and must be part of the food. It is convenient to consider these with the vitamins. A dietary requirement for carbohydrate exists only under the artificial conditions in which protein is restricted and other precursors of glucose (carbohydrate and glycerol) are excluded.

Table 1. Micro- and macro-nutrients contrasted

	Micro-nutrients	Macro-nutrients
1.	Consumed in small amounts (usually <1 g/day)	Large amounts (many g/day)
2.	Absorbed unchanged*	Degraded by digestion
3.	Essential, body cannot make them	No single carbohydrate, fat or protein as eaten is essential but products may be (see text)
4.	Do not provide energy	Provide energy
5.	Major function as coenzymes and catalysts	Enzymes are proteins
6.	Structural function limited (calcium, phosphorus mainly)	Protein mainly structural, but also some lipid and carbohydrate

*Exceptions include carotenoids and folates.

Good nutrition (or nutriture) is a matter of balance, neither too much nor too little. *Malnutrition* is *disordered nutrition of any kind* and may be categorized in a number of ways (Table 2).

Table 2. Classification of malnutrition

1.	Cause:	primary (exogenous)
		secondary (endogenous)
2.	Type:	excess, toxicity (overnutrition)
		deficiency (undernutrition)
3.	Nutrient:	vitamins, elements, protein, energy sources
4.	Degree:	(i) mild – moderate – severe or, alternatively,
		(ii) depleted stores – biochemical lesion – functional change – structural lesion
5.	Duration:	acute, sub-acute, chronic
6.	Outcome:	reversible, irreversible

Part 1 Protein Energy Malnutrition (PEM)

This term is now in common use for all degrees (mild, moderate and severe) and clinical types (marasmus, marasmic-kwashiorkor and kwashiorkor) of the most widespread nutritional disorder of childhood. However, there is no essential difference between inanition in the adult and marasmus in the infant, and kwashiorkor occasionally occurs in adults on diets very low in protein or with impaired protein utilization. It seems justified therefore to use PEM to cover all nutritional disorders in which there is deficiency of protein and energy in any combination and of whatever origin.

Inanition

This denotes a total reduction in the intake of all nutrients amounting to complete starvation in the most severe form. The highest priority is given by the body to the need to meet its energy requirements. If these cannot be met from dietary sources then the body's stores of glycogen and, more importantly, fat are drawn upon. In addition the protein of the lean body mass is also catabolized and the consequent wasting of organs and muscles results.

It is being increasingly recognized that inanition arises not only in populations subjected to famine conditions but also is a frequent complication impairing recovery in surgical patients and those suffering from chronic wasting diseases, in whom food intake is greatly reduced.

1 Cachexia. An extreme example of the loss of muscular and adipose tissue in terminal illness.

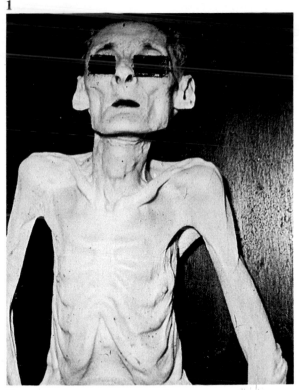

2 Hypercatabolic disease. This occurs in acute illness or injury usually associated with sepsis in which there is an increase in metabolic rate and of net protein catabolism of 25% and more. This 27-year-old patient with ulcerative colitis required an emergency colectomy after losing weight from 44 to 25 kg. After operation the weight continued to fall to 22 kg and normal weight was only regained after 3 months in hospital.

3 Hypercatabolic disease. Posterior view of the same patient.

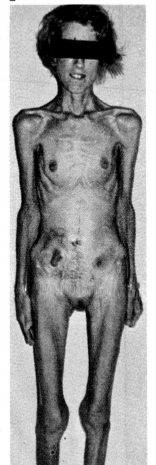

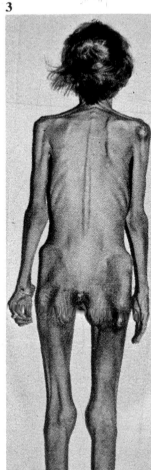

4 Parotid enlargement. There is bilateral, chronic, non-inflammatory swelling of the parotid glands, with no change in the overlying skin. It is usually seen in older children and adults and is an indication of prolonged undernutrition. It has also been reported to occur in chronically starved subjects during refeeding.

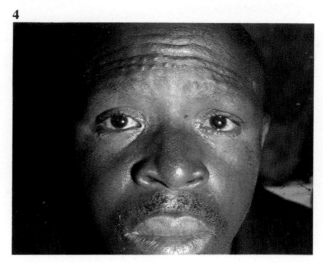

5 Xerotic skin. In chronic undernutrition in adults the skin of the extremities is frequently abnormally dry and superficially fissured. The skin over most of the body is thinned, wrinkled and has lost its usual elasticity; amounting to premature ageing.

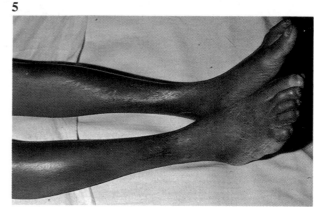

6 Hyperkeratosis. The skin over parts of the body is thickened, dry and wrinkled. The perifollicular areas are sometimes affected, with heaping up of hyperkeratotic material, but this appearance is more especially associated with vitamin A deficiency (**71 & 72**).

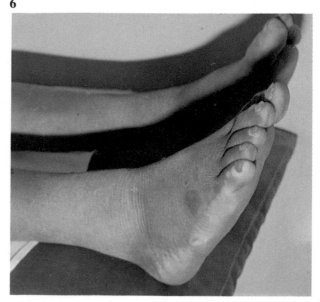

7 'Permanent goose flesh.' This term was given to a condition of the skin commonly seen in chronically undernourished adults by B.S. Platt. It superficially resembles cutis anserina, with prominence of the pilo-sebaceous follicles but they are not frankly keratotic, as in perifollicular hyperkeratosis (**71 & 72**). Its significance remains uncertain.

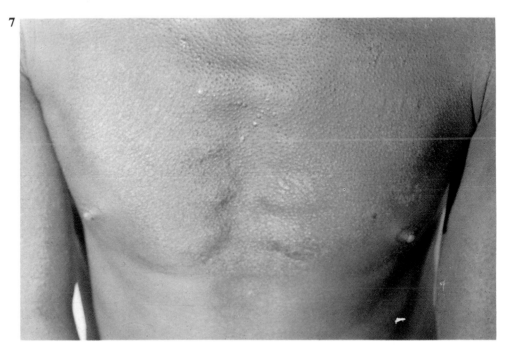

Early PEM in childhood

This is evidenced by growth failure in the pre-clinical stage. Serial measurements of height and weight are important in early detection. Biochemical changes in circulating amino acids and urinary excretion products of protein metabolism precede the development of clinical disease.

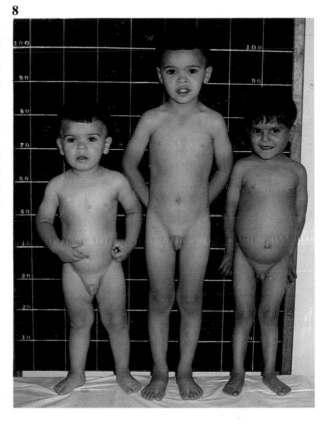

8 Growth failure. The children in this picture were aged 2, 4½ and 5½ years from left to right. The first two are normal but the last is grossly retarded in growth although the weight/height ratio is normal and there is no evidence of clinical malnutrition. Stunting is the commonest evidence of chronic, mild PEM.

9 Growth chart in mild PEM. Supervision and weighing at regular intervals form a useful means of monitoring progress. In this case weaning from the breast was followed by a dramatic fall in weight and frank kwashiorkor was precipitated by an attack of measles, but a good recovery was made.

An apparently satisfactory weight gain may mask a change in body composition towards extracellular fluid retention preceding kwashiorkor, and weight should be related to height. In severe PEM X-rays show transverse lines of bone growth retardation with thinning of bone texture.

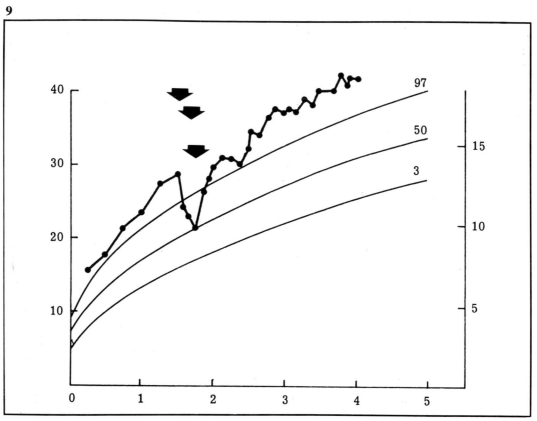

10 Measles in the undernourished child is always a serious disease. The rash often assumes a florid form as in this Guatemalan child. It frequently precipitates overt kwashiorkor (see **27–42**) with a marked fall in serum albumin, and xerophthalmia (see **43–73**). Cell-mediated immunity is markedly impaired.

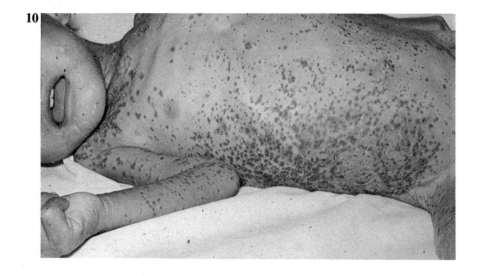

11 Enteritis necroticans (Pigbel) old woman feeding her pig. In the highlands of New Guinea, enteritis necroticans is related to pig feasting which is an integral and complex part of the indigenous culture of the highland tribes. The feeding of infant pigs may even take priority over the feeding of human infants. An interesting, if rare, example of how the 'deposed child' situation can lead to malnutrition.

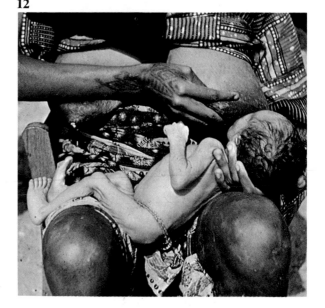

12 Inanition despite adequate lactation. The breasts are engorged and the flattened nipples make sucking difficult. The six week old baby is wasted, weighing only 2¼ kg.

Marasmus

This is wasting (marasmos) in the young child and is due to total reduction in food intake. This commonly results from gastroenteritis of fly-borne infections in the summer and respiratory infections in the winter. The abandonment of breast feeding and resort to artificial feeding of diluted formulae from dirty feeding bottles aggravates the problem. Infants are commonly affected as the associated feeding problems commence at birth or shortly afterwards. It is the predominant form of PEM throughout developing countries and is on the increase as urban slums grow as the result of rapid social change.

13 Extreme wasting in marasmus. This affects all body tissues and the marked loss of subcutaneous fat and skeletal muscle results in a 'skin and bone' appearance. Body weight may be reduced to only 40% or so of the normal mean for age. The prognosis is especially grave in those cases with 50% or more loss of body weight.

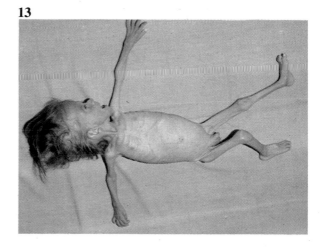

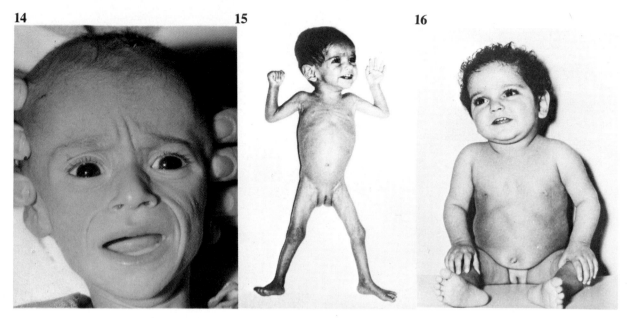

14 **'Monkey' facies.** The wizened, 'old man' appearance of the face with sunken, wrinkled cheeks, is characteristic of prolonged and severe marasmus. In milder cases the normally large buccal fat pads are preserved long after wasting of deeper fat elsewhere.

15 **Severe marasmus before treatment.** There is generalized wasting, and in contrast to kwashiorkor, these infants are extremely hungry.

16   The same patient after 3 months of treatment. A modified cow's milk formula with added arachis or other oil provides a concentrated source of energy. The diet should be introduced step-wise to provide eventually about 200 kcal and 3–5 kg protein/kg/day. Catch-up growth is usually slow during the first month but rapid thereafter.

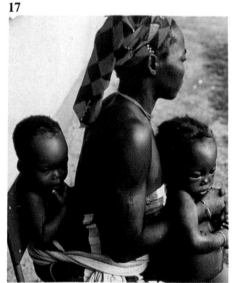

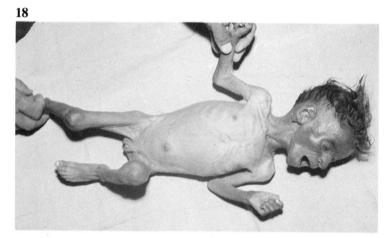

18 **False appearance of 'enlarged joints'.** Marked muscle wasting, as in this 5 month old infant, may mislead the physician into believing that the limb joints are swollen.

17 **Identical twins.** Twins constitute a serious feeding problem in poor communities. They are usually given a special significance; being regarded as lucky by some and unlucky by others. The twin in front of the mother has kwashiorkor.

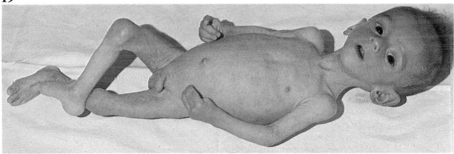

19 Main d'accoucheur. The characteristic contraction of the hands in this marasmic infant is indicative of accompanying tetany. This may be due to calcium deficiency, magnesium deficiency or a combination of both.

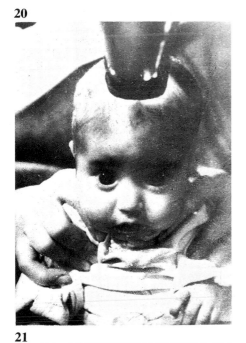

20 Cranial transillumination. Appearance of the skull of a normal child.

21 The appearance of this child with severe marasmus and of that in the next picture with kwashiorkor both contrast markedly with the normal. The brain substance fills the cranium less completely and the skull table is less well outlined. With experience this can form a simple non-invasive test.

22 See above.

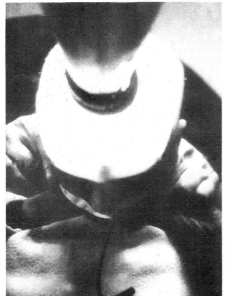

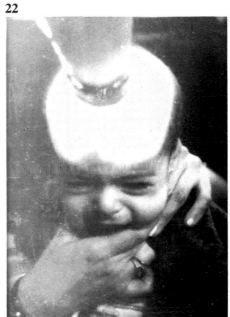

23 Skull in failure to thrive. 2½ year old male hospitalized for failure to thrive. Lateral skull X-ray at time of admission shows no gross abnormalities.

23

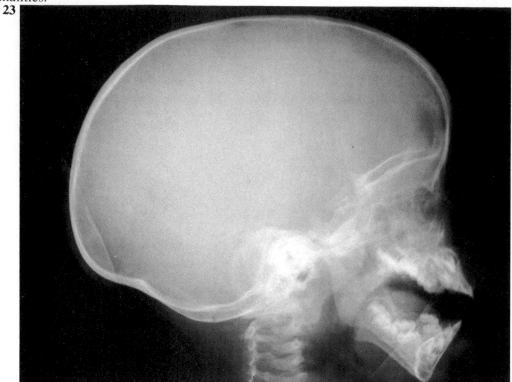

24 Skull in failure to thrive. Two months later when the child had gained weight and was well, the lateral skull X-ray shows wide coronal and lamboid sutures, indicating growth of the brain.

24

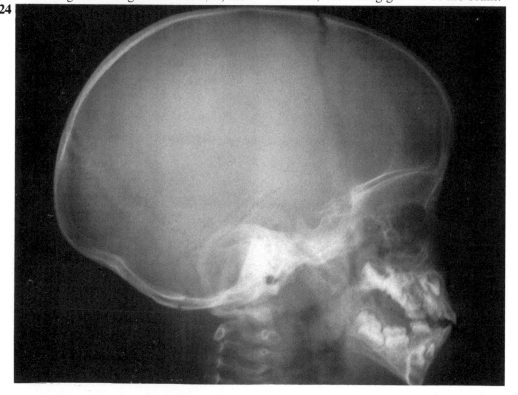

25 Gastro-intestinal tract in marasmus. Gastro-intestinal series 2 weeks after admission demonstrates a large stomach and separate loops of small intestine with thickened valvulae conniventes.

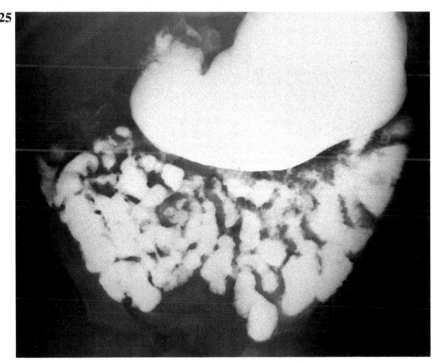

26 Gastro-intestinal tract in marasmus. Four weeks after the original study when the patient was well, a repeat intestinal series shows the small intestine to be normal.

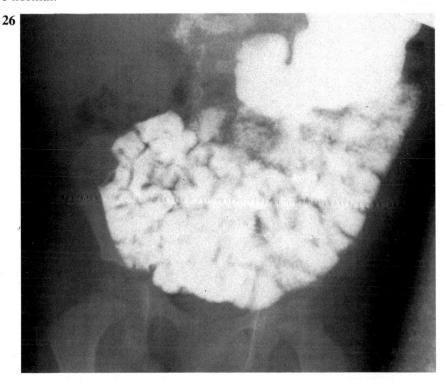

Kwashiorkor

This name has been adopted from the Ga dialect of Ghana where the syndrome, characterized primarily by protein deficiency, was first described. It is the predominant form of childhood malnutrition in those areas where the basic staple is starchy roots like cassava and yam. These are parts of Africa south of the Sahara, and Pacific and Caribbean islands. Children in the second and subsequent years are usually affected as breast feeding, often prolonged, together with starchy supplementary foods, fails to meet the protein requirements of the growing child.

27

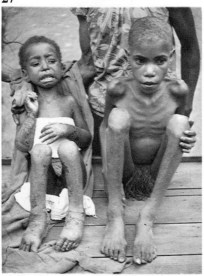

27 Kwashiorkor and marasmus in brothers. Compare the miserable expression, pale hair, generalized oedema and skin changes in the child on the left with the marasmic wasting of his older brother. Kwashiorkor frequently follows acute infection and/or diarrhoea in a child during the weaning period. Some have speculated that this might occur because of genetic differences, involving in particular the endocrine system. It seems more reasonable to suppose that, just as the same child may go through various phases and forms of malnutrition, so siblings might be exposed to somewhat different diets and other predisposing factors within the family, which is itself a constantly changing micro-environment.

28

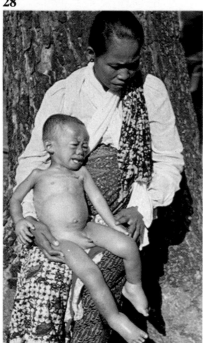

29

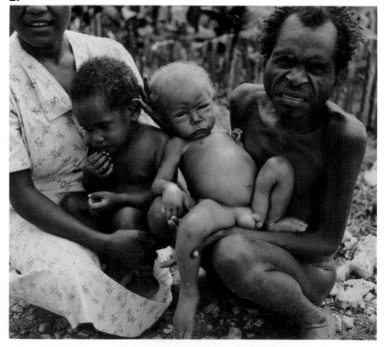

28 Typical kwashiorkor. This Indonesian child shows marked oedema, mental changes and sparse, light coloured hair, which contrasts with that of the mother.

29 De-pigmentation in kwashiorkor. The contrast with the normal child is striking; a tribe in New Guinea.

30 Kwashiorkor and marasmus.
Contrasted appearance at postmortem. The child on the left with kwashiorkor has generalized oedema, preservation of subcutaneous fat and gross enlargement of the liver with fatty infiltration. In marasmus (right) there is no oedema, muscle and fat are wasted, and the liver is shrunken.

30

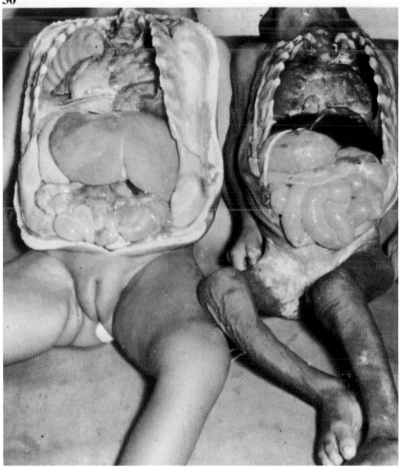

32 Oedema of the hands in kwashiorkor. The occurrence of oedema is related to hypoalbuminaemia and impaired renal function leading to increased sodium retention.

31

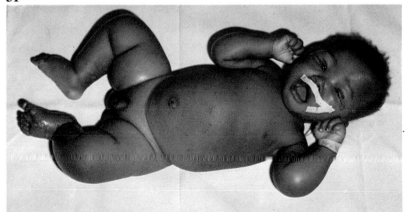

32

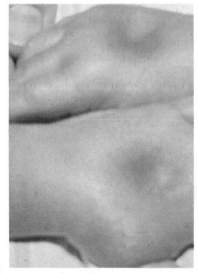

31 'Sugar baby.' This term was first used for the severe form of kwashiorkor commonly seen in Jamaica and attributed to a high sugar, and consequently very low protein, diet. Marked oedema, fatty liver and low serum albumin are the main features and skin changes are absent or minimal. This is a Bantu baby in Johannesburg.

33 Dermatosis of kwashiorkor. This is one of the most characteristic features and is absent in marasmus. There is increased pigmentation with a tendency to desquamation leaving hypopigmented skin and superficial ulceration and the liability to secondary infection. Confluent areas have been termed 'flaky-paint' or 'crazy-paving' dermatosis, and small lesions 'enamel spots'. The skin on most parts of the body may be involved, especially the buttocks, inner thighs and perineum, but the photo-sensitive areas affected in pellagra (**84–90**) are spared. Although characteristic of kwashiorkor the lesion has been wrongly attributed to burns or scalds. A careful history and general examination will readily lead to a correct diagnosis.

33

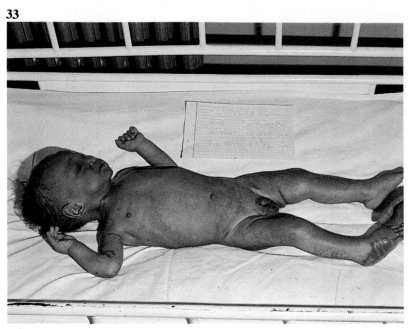

34 The skin in the flexures of the legs is especially liable to become dirty, soggy and devitalized and so subject to peeling.

34

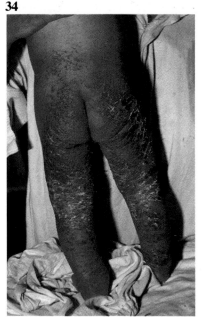

35 Hyperpigmentation in a fair skin. In contrast to the frequent depigmentation in the dark-skinned, kwashiorkor skin changes are less marked in those with a fair skin and sometimes consist of hyperpigmentation. This characteristically occurs on the forehead as in this Jordanian child.

35

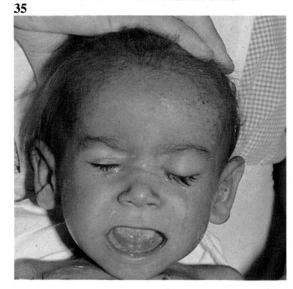

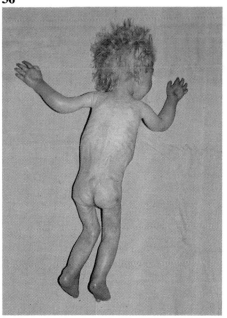

36

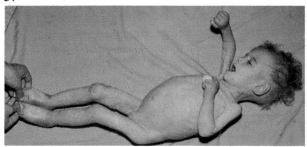

36 **Marasmic-kwashiorkor.** Many children with PEM, as this Jordanian child, show features of marasmus (emaciation) and of kwashiorkor (oedema of the hands and legs).

37 **Marasmic-kwashiorkor.** In many areas this is the most common form of kwashiorkor and tends to have a better prognosis than the full-blown form.

37

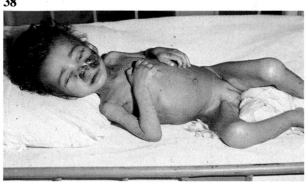

38

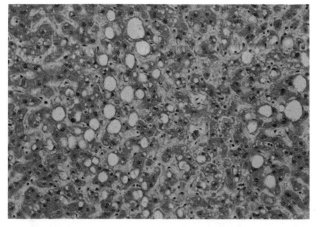

38 **Noma in kwashiorkor.** This severely malnourished young Egyptian child has the uncommon complication to kwashiorkor of noma (cancrum oris) (see **280 & 281**). Keratomalacia was also present in both eyes (one is shown in **62**).

39

39 **Fatty liver in kwashiorkor.** This is one of the most typical findings in the disease and is not seen in marasmus, in which the liver is shrunken. Small fat droplets appear first in the peripheral area of the liver lobule and spread progressively to the central vein area with coalescence to form large globules. With treatment the fat disappears in the reverse order. There is proliferation of reticulin fibres radiating from the portal tract but cirrhosis does not result, in contrast to the fatty liver in alcoholism (**264 & 265**).

40 Moon face. This is seen usually in those cases of kwashiorkor with marked oedema of the extremities and lumbar region. It subsides rapidly with treatment. The emaciated, 'monkey' facies of marasmus (**14**) should be contrasted with it. Moon face is also seen in chronic ankylostomiasis with severe anaemia; rare in preschool children. Unlike the moon face of obesity (**228**) it is not due to excess deposition of fat. In hypercorticolism there is often erythema.

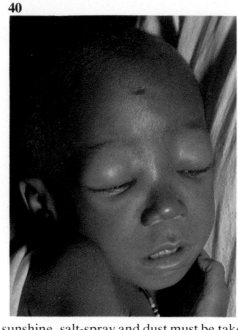

40

41 Hair changes. These are a constant feature of kwashiorkor but may also be seen in marasmus. The hair is dull and dry and lacks its normal lustre. It is finer and more silky in texture than normal and sparse – covering the scalp less abundantly and with wider spaces between hairs. Naturally long hair is unusually straight, untidy and 'staring'. In black children the thick, tight, short curls become unruly and straightened. Hairs become loose and are readily plucked out. Normally black hair becomes greyish or reddish in colour – dyschromotrichia; but local factors such as dyeing, the effect of sunshine, salt-spray and dust must be taken into account.

42 The 'flag-sign' or signa de bandera. This was first described from Costa Rica. When the hair is long and naturally dark, as in this child in El Salvador, it may show alternating darker and lighter bands when held up, corresponding respectively to periods of better and poor nutrition. Under a dissecting microscope deformities in the hair root bulb can be detected quite early on, and the appearances differ in marasmus and kwashiorkor.

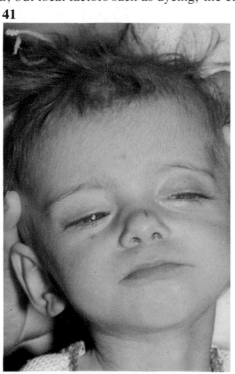

41

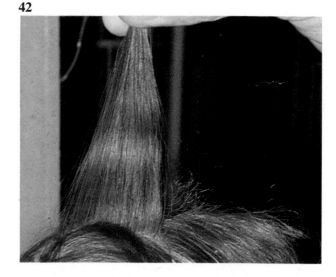

42

Part 2 Vitamin Deficiency, Toxicity and Dependency

Vitamin deficiencies may occur as a result of inadequate dietary intake or secondarily from impaired absorption or some other stage in the utilization of the vitamin. Toxicity arises from prolonged excessive intake or very high dosing with a vitamin. It is confined to the fat-soluble vitamins A, D and K that are stored in high concentration in the body.

Vitamin dependency is a state of impaired cellular metabolism in which the coenzyme form of a vitamin is present in normal concentration but coupling to the apoenzyme is defective. This may arise either as a result of chemical interference with the availability of the coenzyme to the apoenzyme, or because of a genetic defect in one enzyme or more involved in this reaction. Vitamin dependency is known to occur in relation to pyridoxine, vitamin B_{12} and biotin (**128 & 129**).

Vitamin A (Retinol)

The daily requirement of about 750 μg is normally met about equally from animal sources of the preformed vitamin and active carotenoids from vegetables. Large amounts are normally stored in the liver, except in the young child in whom deficiency most commonly occurs.

The WHO has introduced a classification of xerophthalmia and this is used here in illustrating the various stages (XIA etc.).

43

44

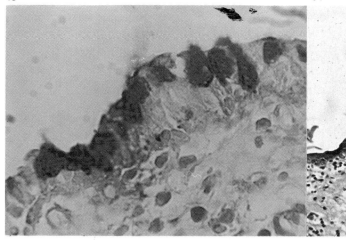

Vitamin A deficiency

45

43 Conjunctival histology in xerophthalmia. The very thin epithelium is desquamating and consists of keratinized cell layers with flattened nuclei. The basal cell layer retains the ability to regenerate normal epithelium once vitamin A is supplied. (H&E, ×100)

44 Conjunctival histology of healing xerophthalmia. The epithelium is still only one or two cells thick. There are now numerous mucus-secreting goblet cells. (PAS & AB, ×400)

45 Normal cornea. This section shows the normal appearance of basal, wing and squamous epithelial cells. Many keratocytes are found in the anterior stroma.(×500)

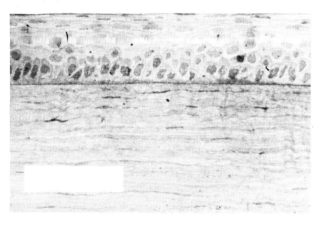

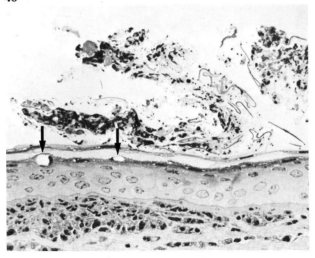

46 Vitamin A deficient cornea. After 6 weeks of experimental deficiency in the rat the columnar appearance of the basal epithelium is lost, with keratinizing epithelium at the surface. There is accumulation of keratin, inflammatory cells, and amorphous cellular debris. Two cysts (arrows) are located in the superficial epithelial layers. (×500)

47 Normal conjunctiva. The epithelium shows three or four layers of cells with goblet cells (arrows) interspersed. (×500, inset ×1000)

48 Vitamin A deficient conjunctiva. There is superficial keratinization of the epithelium, loss of goblet cells, and rite peg formation (arrows) where the thickness is twice normal. (×500)

47

48

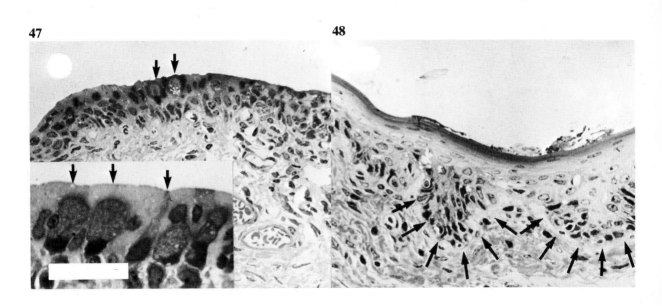

49 Early conjunctival xerosis (X1A). Dryness and unwettability of the conjunctival surface are characteristic of this early stage of vitamin A deficiency. Wrinkling and increased pigmentation may also be present, as in this case, but are not on their own an indication of vitamin A deficiency. Plasma vitamin A was 9 μg/100 ml (normal 20–50 μg/100 ml). Evidence of night blindness can be elicited by careful history taking and observation of the behaviour of the young child at dusk even at this early stage.

49

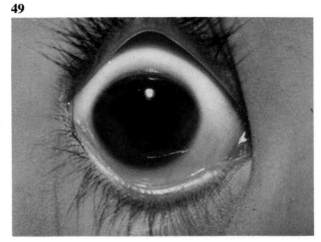

50 Bitot's spots (X1B). These are single or, as in this case, multiple areas of desquamated, keratinized conjunctival cells together with lipid material from the Meibomian glands. They are not pathognomonic of vitamin A deficiency, as sometimes supposed, but only of nutritional aetiology if accompanied by conjunctival xerosis, as here.

51 A large, diffuse, foamy Bitot's spot. Bitot's original description in 1868 mentioned 'Particles arranged in a series of wavy parallel lines, which give the lesion the appearance of an undulating and rippled surface'. *Corynebacterium xerosis* can usually be grown from these lesions and it has been suggested that this gas-forming organism is responsible for the bubbles that give the foamy appearance.

50

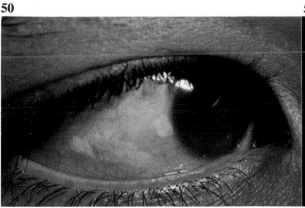

51

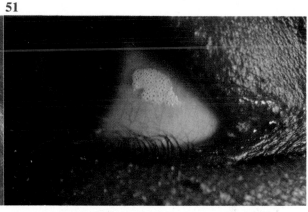

52 A large, compact Bitot's spot. This is a less common appearance than the foamy lesion (**50 & 51**), in which the desquamated epithelial material is more dense and has a 'cheesy' appearance. The 'cheesy' lesion appears to be more chronic than the 'foamy' and those that occur in older children and may be stigmata of previous vitamin A deficiency are often of this kind. Under these circumstances they do not respond to vitamin A treatment.

52

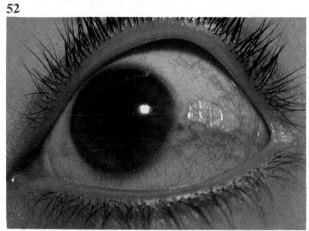

53 Nasally situated Bitot's spot. This is rare compared with the temporal position. The reason is unclear. It has been suggested that exposure, a factor thought to play a part in the accumulation of Bitot's spot material, is less on the nasal side. Another theory is that the lids are less closely applied on the nasal side and therefore less likely to mould desquamating epithelial cells into a spot.

53

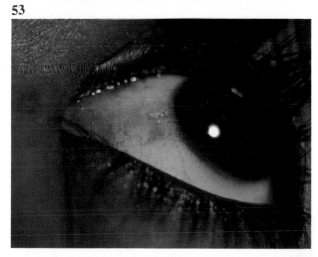

54 Bitot's spot related to ectropion. Light is thrown on the aetiology of Bitot's spot by this and other rare instances in the literature of material accumulating on part of the conjunctiva not normally exposed to the atmosphere. That exposure does play a part, possibly by creating instability of the tear film covering the conjunctiva, is also borne out by the fact that Bitot's spots are often confined to the normally exposed inter-palpebral area of the conjunctiva, or if more extensive most of the material accumulates there.

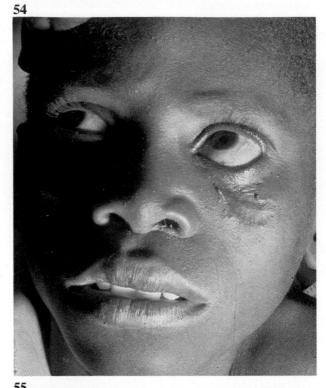

55 Extensive Bitot's spot material involving cornea and conjunctiva. Bitot's spots are usually confined to the conjunctiva even when quite extensive. Rarely xerosis and desquamation also affect the cornea, especially if the process is very low grade and chronic, as in this Jordanian child. There was no corneal ulceration or keratomalacia and complete clearing occurred with vitamin A therapy.

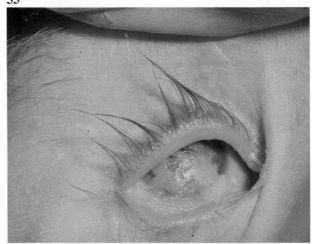

56 Measles kerato-conjunctivitis and xeroph-thalmia. There is xerosis of the conjunctiva stained with 1% rose bengal. Attributable to measles are the slight chemosis, minimal conjunctival infection and corneal erosions stained with 1% fluorescein.

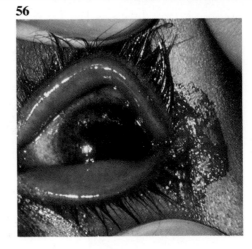

57 Measles kerato-conjunctivitis and xerophthalmia. The corneal light reflex is distorted and the pre-ocular tear film is lacking.

58 Conjunctival histology in measles. This should be contrasted with the histological appearance in xerophthalmia (**43 & 44**). The epithelium is thickened and hypoplastic and the cells are swollen and have pyknotic nuclei. There is giant cell formation (as in parts of the respiratory tract) and goblet cells are lacking. (H&E, ×100)

57

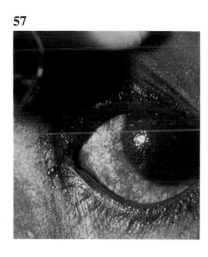

58

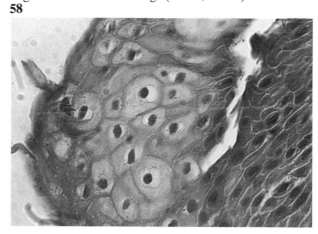

59 Marked conjunctival xerosis with corneal xerosis (X1A and X2). The conjunctiva is very dry, thickened and thrown into numerous folds. The cornea is also dry, has lost its normal lustre and its stroma is infiltrated with white cells. From the limbic plexus there is early invasion of the corneal substance by capillaries (neovascularization). There is a superficial erosion situated below the pupillary area, but this has not breached the continuity of the epithelium and has not reached the stage of 'ulceration' (see **60**). Plasma vitamin A was only 3 μg/dl (normal 20–50 μg/dl).

60 Corneal 'ulceration' with xerosis (X3A). This is the earliest change in which an irreversible element occurs; some degree of scarring is inevitable. Mucin deficiency in the tears as a result of atrophy of conjunctival goblet cells causes instability of the pre-corneal film and the 'break-up time' (BUT) is shortened to less than 10 seconds. Ulceration does not imply infection in this context and xerosis of the cornea is a constant feature. It involves loss of substance of a part or of the whole of the corneal thickness. Minimal denudation of the epithelial surface (erosion) without transgression of Bowman's membrane leaves no permanent damage and is not included in this stage. When the ulcer progresses to advanced stromal loss it may result in descemetocele or complete perforation with iris prolapse.

59

60

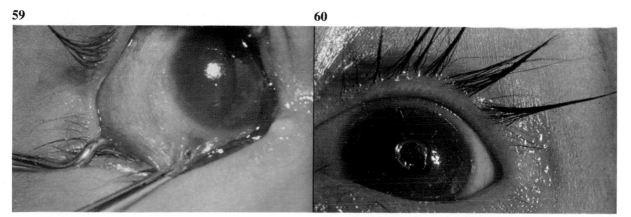

61 Keratomalacia – typical appearance (X3B).
Although any part or all of the cornea may be
affected, the central area as shown here is most
commonly affected when the patient is first seen.
Even with prompt vitamin A treatment gross
scarring will be inevitable. The precise nature of
the pathological process that leads to dissolution
of the cornea – termed colliquative necrosis – is not
understood. It bears a resemblance to that seen in
alkali burns of the cornea. It is probable that
instability of the pre-corneal film and keratinization
of epithelial cells lead to activation of corneal
collagenase and/or other proteases, resulting in
liquefaction.

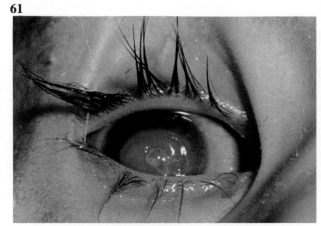

62 Keratomalacia – total (X3B). This is the
appearance of one eye of the child in **38**. In the
other eye the process was not quite so advanced
but sight was also destroyed. The entire thickness
of the whole of the cornea is a cloudy, gelatinous
mass. Particularly in very young children, keratomalacia may develop very rapidly and, as in this
case, there may be complete absence of xerosis and
Bitot's spot formation in the conjunctiva. The
minimal reaction in the surrounding tissues and
lack of discharge are characteristic and assist in the
differentiation from other conditions.

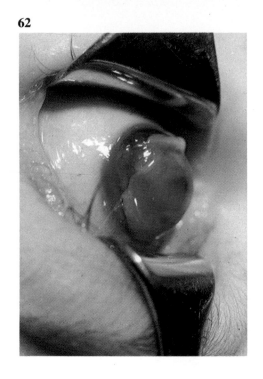

63 Keratomalacia with prolapse of the lens. A
serious complication which leads to disorganization
of the eye contents and subsequent blindness. The
total lack of inflammatory reaction is remarkable
but characteristic.

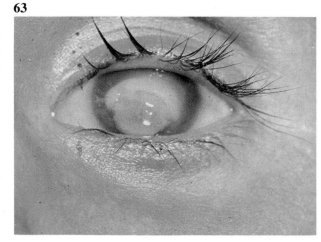

64 Panophthalmitis. Perforation of the cornea in keratomalacia frequently leads to the introduction of secondary infection and destruction of the eye. Fortunately this often occurs in only one eye and useful vision may be preserved in the other with prompt vitamin A therapy.

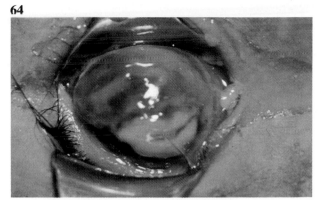

65 Ectasia of the cornea (XS). During the active stage the softened cornea has bulged forwards before the intra-ocular pressure. The scar usually consists of a thick epithelial layer lying upon scar tissue that is thinner than the normal stroma. As is the case for all corneal scars, a diagnosis of previous xerophthalmia can only be presumptive, and based on a careful history (**67**).

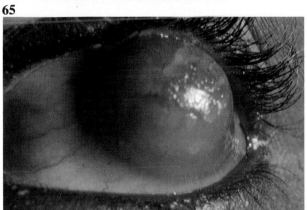

66 Anterior staphyloma (XS). The extensive corneal defect has been stretched before the scar tissue has consolidated and the wound has been complicated by the incorporation of corneal tissue.

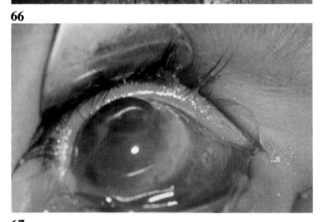

67 Corneal scars (XS). These are of varying density; very fine (nebula), moderately dense (macula) and very dense (leucoma). They also vary in size, from pin-head, to involvement of the entire cornea. The cornea may be scarred from many causes besides previous vitamin A deficiency, including injury and many kinds of eye infection. As they tend to be of higher prevalence than active lesions in communities subject to vitamin A deficiency it is important to distinguish those of nutritional aetiology if possible. A history of the onset of the eye lesions between about 2 months and 5 years of age accompanying general malnutrition is suggestive. Absence of injury, prolonged purulent discharge or severe trachoma in the history supports the likelihood of vitamin A deficiency as the cause. Both corneas are likely to be affected to some degree, and if only part of the cornea is scarred it is frequently the inferior central area that is affected as in this Syrian infant.

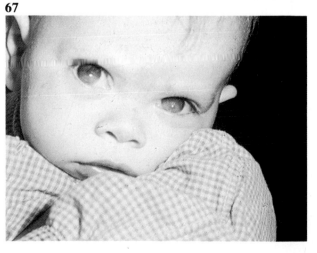

68 Adherent leucoma (XS). The corneal changes have been arrested before perforation but the iris has become adherent to the cornea and the pupil is distorted behind a dense disc-shaped leucoma.

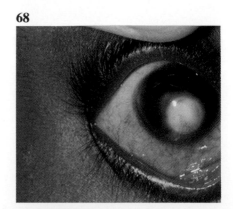

69 Adherent leucoma with anterior polar cataract (XS). The lens is otherwise clear and the pupil is not distorted. The small, dense leucoma is inferiorly situated and some useful vision will be retained.

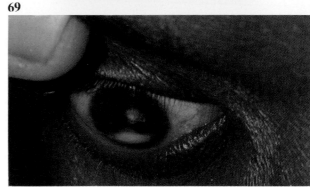

70 Xerophthalmia fundus (XF). Fundus photograph shows the characteristic whitish speckled appearance of the affected retina. Fluorescein angiography revealed 'window' defects which appeared to be in the pigment epithelium. The appearance cleared with vitamin A therapy but some of the window defects remained. Retinitis punctata albescens and fundus albi punctatus are very similar in appearance but do not respond to treatment. Fundus changes are a rare manifestation of vitamin A deficiency and have only been reported from areas of high endemicity, as in Indonesia.

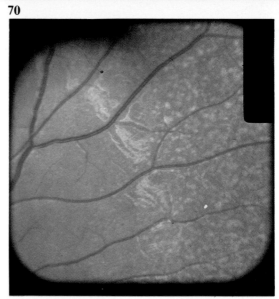

71 Perifollicular hyperkeratosis (phrynoderma, toad skin). Spinous papules appear at the tips of the hair follicles against the background of a generally dry and rough skin. Areas first affected are the postero-lateral parts of the arm (as in this case) and the antero-lateral aspects of the thighs. There is steady spread to the extensor surfaces of the limbs, shoulders and lower part of abdomen. The chest, back and buttocks are usually only involved in very extensive cases. It is only seen in undernourished subjects and has most frequently been associated with vitamin A deficiency and general undernourishment. It is easily differentiated from the perifollicular haemorrhages of scurvy (137). Ichthyosis is familial and affects the entire skin. Keratosis pilaris is similar but occurs in well nourished adolescents. Acne vulgaris has a different distribution and features pustulation. Perifollicular hyperkeratosis is not seen before school age.

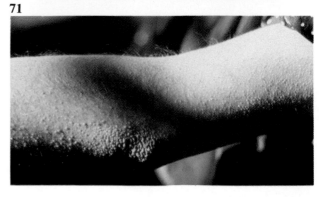

72 Perifollicular hyperkeratosis. The shin is a common site as in this Turkoman child.

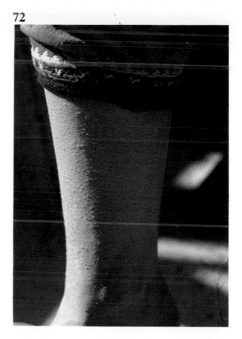

73 Dermomalacia. This was the name given by Pillat to the liquefactive skin changes he observed in severely vitamin A-deficient Chinese soldiers in the 1930s. The gross hyperkeratinization of the skin surrounding the eyes in this infant with severe keratomalacia is an early stage of the condition and is a rare occurrence.

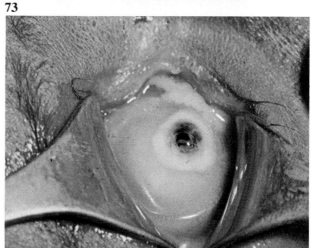

Vitamin A toxicity

74 Hypervitaminosis A. Acute toxicity causes nausea, vomiting and headache due to raised intracranial pressure (pseudotumour cerebri) and peeling of the skin. Chronic poisoning results in loss of weight, low-grade fever, tenderness over the long bones and skull changes (see below) and a pruritic rash. Bright red marginal discolouration of the gingiva as shown here is characteristic.

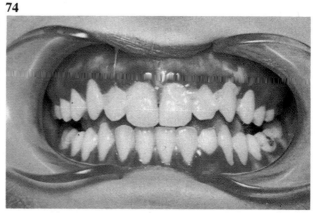

75 Skull in hypervitaminosis A. Frontal view of a 2 year old female showing wide sagittal and coronal sutures.

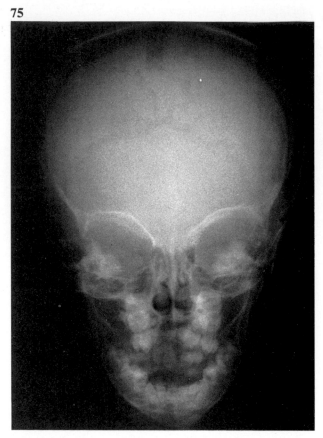

75

76 Skull in hypervitaminosis A. Lateral view of the same case.

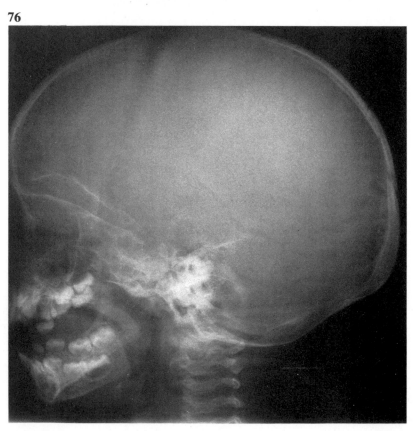

76

77 Hypercarotenosis. Prolonged excessive ingestion of carotenoids in carrot juice, carrots or dark green leafy vegetables leads to high blood levels and staining of the whole body. The condition is benign and subsides after withdrawal of the source. It may occur secondarily in diabetes mellitus, hypothyroidism or anorexia nervosa.

77

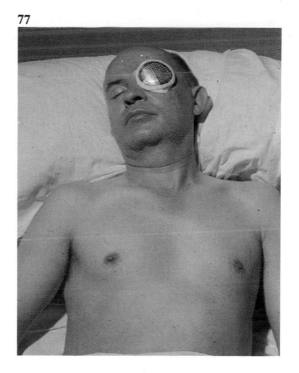

78 Hypercarotenosis. The face, eye and palm of the hand. The sclerae remain clear, distinguishing the condition from jaundice.

79 Hypercarotenosis. The sole of the foot. The staining is usually heaviest on the palms and soles due to the secretion of carotenoids by sebaceous glands heavily concentrated in these areas.

78

79

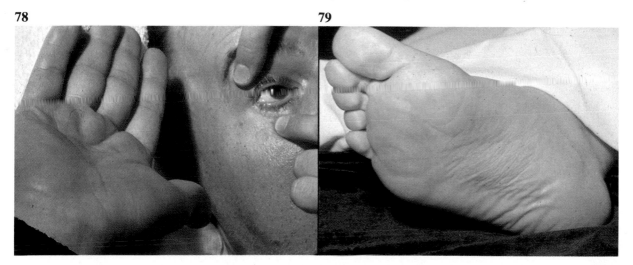

Thiamin (Vitamin B₁)

Many dietaries barely meet the daily requirement of about 1 mg. Prolonged cooking causes loss, and in chronic alcoholism absorption is impaired and requirements increased for thiamin pyrophosphate a coenzyme in carbohydrate metabolism.

A rare genetic degenerative disorder, Leigh's disease or necrotizing encephalopathy is thought to be due to a defect in thiamin metabolism.

80 Wrist drop and foot drop. This patient has chronic polyneuritic 'dry' beriberi. In these patients there is also loss of tendon reflexes, joint position sense, and vibration sense, tenderness in the calf muscles on pressure, anaesthesia of the skin especially over the tibia, paraesthesia in the legs and arms and motor weakness.

81 'Wet' or cardiac beriberi. Generalized oedema results from biventricular heart failure with pulmonary congestion. Peripheral vasodilatation, mainly in skeletal muscle, leads to high output failure with increased right ventricular pressure and left ventricular filling pressure. Pyruvate and lactate are important substrates for oxidation in cardiac muscle, and the decarboxylation of pyruvate and its subsequent oxidation in the citric acid cycle are blocked in thiamin deficiency. X-ray shows generalized cardiomegaly and pulmonary vascular congestion which rapidly subside in response to bed rest and intravenous thiamin.

80

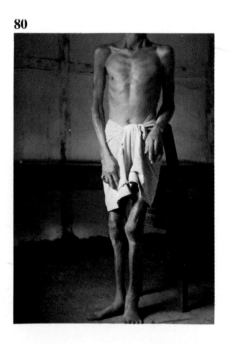

81

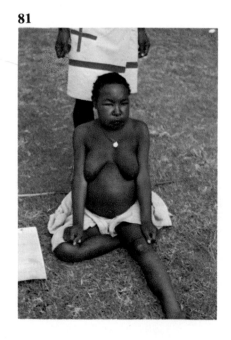

82 Wernicke-Korsakoff syndrome. Mental confusion, aphonia and nystagmus progress to bilateral 6th nerve paralysis and coma. Polyneuropathy is frequent. Aphonia, polyneuropathy and cardiac failure are characteristic of infantile beriberi. This section shows symmetrical haemorrhages in the corpora quadrigemina. Small petechiae are also present in the peri-aqueductal gray matter. (H&E, ×4).

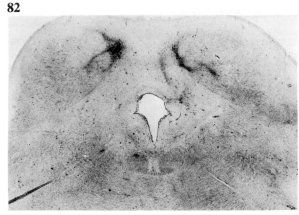

83 Wernicke's encephalopathy. Spongy degeneration in the mamillary body, with loss of nerve cells and astrocytic reaction. Some macrophages contain haemosiderin as the acute haemorrhagic stage is past. (H&E, ×160)

Niacin (Nicotinic acid)

The daily requirement is normally provided from the diet (about 20 mg) and by synthesis from tryptophan in the body. Communities subsisting on maize, the protein of which is deficient in tryptophan, and in which niacin is in an unavailable form are susceptible to pellagra. Lime treatment in the preparation of tortillas releases the niacin and prevents deficiency occurring.

Pellagra may also occur secondary to disturbance of niacin metabolism in Hartnup disease (**252**), treatment with isoniazid and in malignant carcinoid tumour.

84 Early pellagra affecting the arms. The dermatosis begins as an erythema with pruritus and burning. Blebs may run together to form bullae and burst. At the slightly later stage shown the skin becomes hard, rough, cracked, blackish and brittle. In the dark skinned, as in this young Tanzanian male, the dermatosis may be easily overlooked. The symmetrical distribution on parts of the body exposed to the sun is characteristic but lesions are not necessarily confined to these areas. In this case the only other hyperpigmented areas were over those parts of the toes rubbed by ill-fitting shoes.

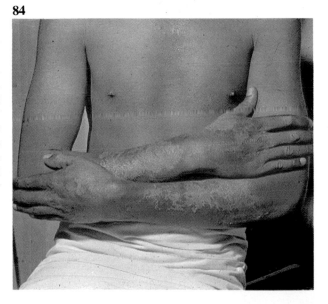

85 Casal's necklace. This fairly broad band or collar of dermatosis running right round the neck, and sometimes extending downwards like a bib, is a classic sign of pellagra. Other parts of the body exposed to the sun are usually also affected.

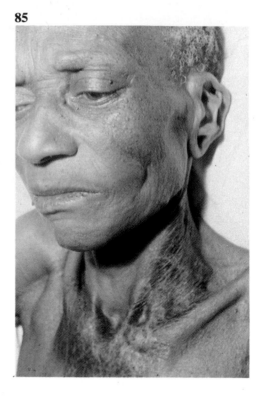

85

86 Extensive pellagrous dermatosis. The symmetrical involvement of the exposed parts of the body and the clear demarcation of the lesions from the normal skin on unexposed parts are striking in this elderly African female patient. It is not clear why the face is frequently unaffected.

86

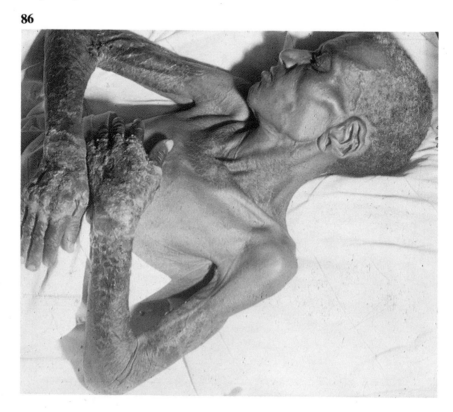

87 Dermatosis of pellagra. The symmetrically equal involvement of the skin of the legs is quite characteristic.   **87**

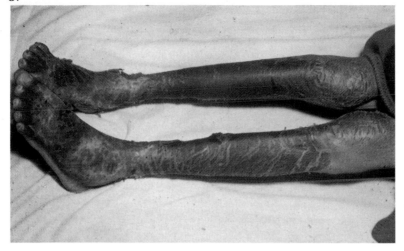

88

88 Dermatosis of pellagra. The backs of the hands and fingers are often the most severely involved parts of the body. The lesions are healing here and the dead skin is being exfoliated.

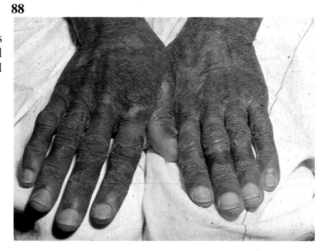

89

89 Chapped cheeks. This roughening and hyper-pigmentation is sometimes mistaken for pellagra. Account should be taken of the influence of exposure, and examination of the classical sites for pellagra will serve to differentiate.

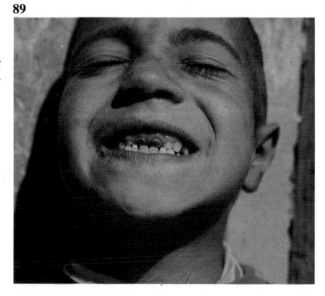

90 Symmetrical chapping of dorsum of hands. This is a common site for the skin changes of pellagra to occur. A careful history and full examination will permit the distinction to be made.

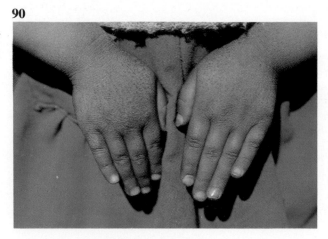

91 Scarlet tongue. The tongue in pellagra is frequently scarlet in appearance and extremely painful. However, this may occur in many non-nutritional conditions and other signs, especially those in the skin, have to be present to make the clinical diagnosis. Fissuring of the tongue alone is not of significance.

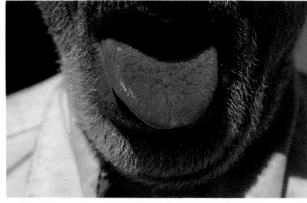

92 Filiform papillary atrophy. This is often seen in deficiency of niacin, folic acid, vitamin B_{12} or iron. It sometimes occurs in well nourished people wearing dentures. The filiform papillae are low or absent, giving a smooth or slick appearance, which remains after scraping lightly with an applicator stick.

93 Fungiform papillary hypertrophy. The condition can be seen and felt as a tongue blade is drawn lightly over the anterior two-thirds of the tongue. Hyperaemia may give the tongue a berry-like appearance. The condition is non-specific and may be due to general undernutrition.

92
93

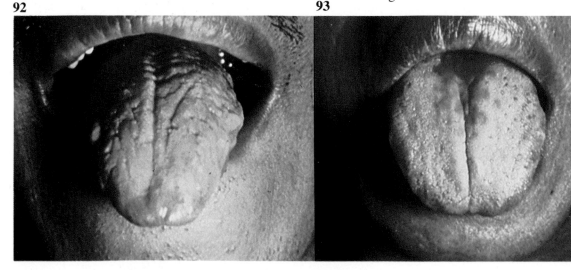

94 Encephalopathy of pellagra. In the late stages this is identical with that of Wernicke (**82 & 83**), but responds to niacin. Early features are depression, apprehension, insomnia, headache and dizziness. Later, tremulous movements or rigidity of the limbs increase and finally, loss of tendon reflexes and numbness and paresis of the limbs progressively incapacitate the patient. The skin changes of pellagra, as in this patient, assist in the differential diagnosis.

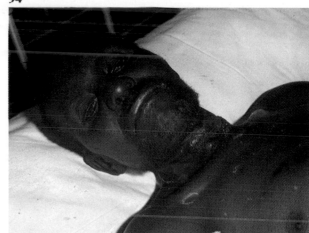

Riboflavin

Many dietaries fail to provide the daily requirement of about 1.5 mg but severe deficiency of this coenzyme, involved in many oxidation-reduction reactions essential to life, is unknown and presumably deficiency is only marginal. This is reflected in the muco-cutaneous lesions pictured here, sometimes collectively known as the 'oro-oculo-genital syndrome'.

95 Magenta tongue. The purplish-red colouration of the tongue, as in this child, is generally regarded as being characteristic of riboflavin deficiency. The tongue is usually sore but other morphologic changes are usually absent.

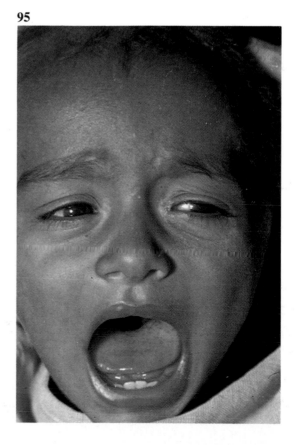

95

96 Tongue in riboflavin deficiency. The patient was an inn-keeper who presented with a number of the features of chronic alcoholism. His main complaint, however, was his very sore tongue, which is seen to be markedly swollen and oedematous and to have a light magenta colour.

97 The same patient as in the previous figure with the tongue returned to its normal size and colour and painless several weeks after large doses of vitamin B complex were administered.

96 **97**

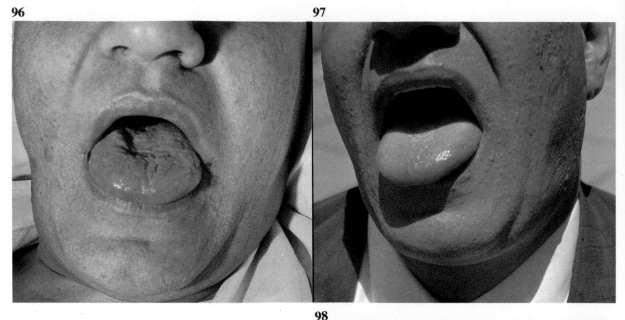

98 Glossitis. A painful and inflamed tongue may occur in other nutritional deficiency states besides pellagra; most notably of riboflavin, folic acid, vitamin B12, pyridoxine or iron. The filiform papillae are atrophic and the fungiform papillae hypertrophic. The differential diagnosis includes uraemia, diabetes mellitus, antibiotic administration, monilial infection, aphthous stomatitis and malignancy. Moeller's glossitis appears as circular, sharply demarcated, denuded areas and is transitory.

98

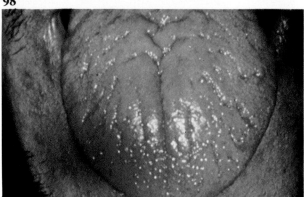

99 Geographic tongue. There are irregularly distributed patchy areas of denudation and atrophy of the epithelium. It is painless and symptomless. The aetiology is obscure, there is no evidence that nutritional factors are involved and it should not be attributed to deficiency of riboflavin or other members of the B vitamin complex.

99

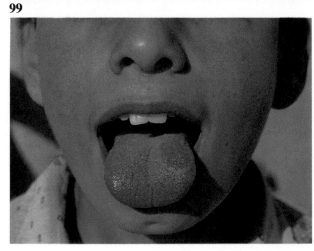

100 Geographic tongue. This patchy denudation of the tongue is often, wrongly, attributed to riboflavin deficiency. It is of no nutritional significance.

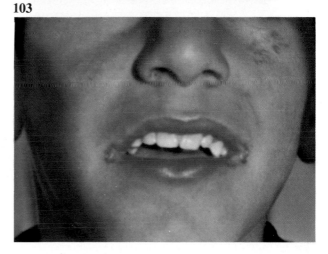

101 Angular stomatitis. The muco-cutaneous junctions at the angles of the mouth are sodden, macerated and excavated with fissuring. Both angles are affected but often unequally. On healing angular scars or rhagades occur (**103**) and must be differentiated from those that follow congenital syphilis. Besides riboflavin deficiency it may also occur in other B vitamin deficiencies and in iron deficiency. Ill-fitting dentures may be responsible. The angles of the eyelids may also be affected – angular palpebritis.

102 Perlèche. In cases of neglect the lesions of angular stomatitis may be colonized by *Candida albicans* giving rise to an exuberant yellowish growth of fungal material. The muco-cutaneous junction of the nose is similarly affected in this young child.

103 Rhagades. Chronic erosions and scarring at the angles of the mouth in a schoolboy in the northeast of Iran where widespread riboflavin deficiency has recently been demonstrated biochemically.

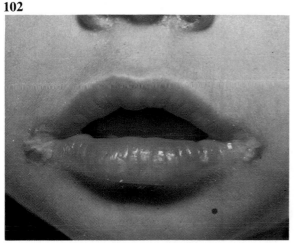

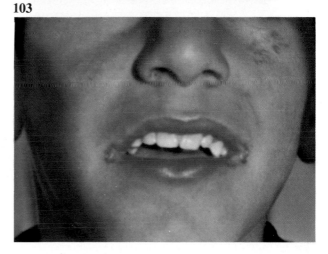

104 Cheilosis. This term should be reserved for vertical fissuring, later complicated by redness, swelling and ulceration of the lips, other than the angles. The centre of the lower lip is usually most affected. Climatic factors, such as cold and wind, may sometimes be responsible.

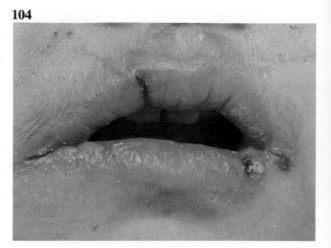

105 Experimental riboflavin deficiency. Early phase of scrotal dermatitis after 175 days on diet that provided 0.51 mg riboflavin per day.

106 More severe lesion of scrotum observed in another patient after 288 days on diet that provided 0.55 mg riboflavin per day. There was no appreciable healing of this lesion until riboflavin supplementation was provided 21 days later.

107 Demonstrates recovery of the same scrotum as that in the previous figure 7 days after the subject was supplemented with 6 mg of riboflavin per day.

105

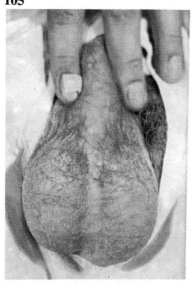

106

107

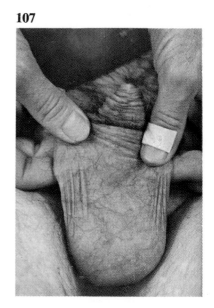

108 **Dyssebacia (shark skin).** The lesion consists of greasy, filiform excrescences, greyish or yellowish-white in colour, most commonly situated on the naso-labial folds, but also occurring on the bridge of the nose, eyebrows and backs of the ears. It is produced by plugging of the enlarged sebaceous glands by retained inspissated sebum.

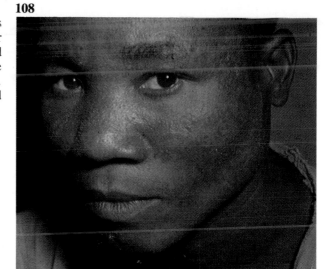

109 **Extreme dyssebacia of the face.** There is also corneal infiltration and early corneal vascularization. This alcoholic African patient also had multiple peripheral neuropathy. A combined vitamin B complex deficiency was suspected in this patient but the lesions shown were most likely to have been due to riboflavin deficiency.

109

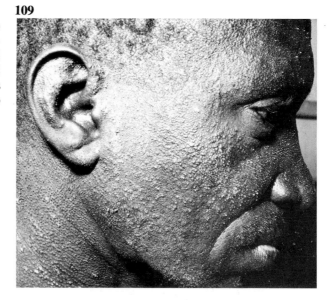

110 The same patient as in the previous figure after 10 days on a good diet and B complex therapy. There is considerable improvement.

110

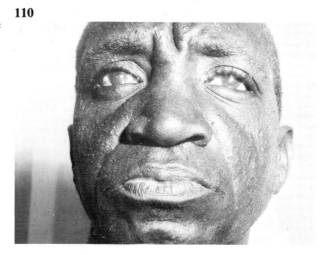

Pyridoxine (Vitamin B₆)

Most diets supply more than the 2 mg required daily. Several rare pyridoxine dependency syndromes have been described including cystathioninuria, homocystinuria (**255 & 256**), familial xanthurenic aciduria and a pyridoxine-responsive anaemia. Treatment necessitates the daily administration of many times the normal infant requirement of about 0.25 mg. Convulsions and abnormal electro-encephalographic recordings have been reported in infants fed a formula in which pyridoxine had been destroyed by heat treatment. Dramatic response occurred when pyridoxine was administered.

111 Pyridoxine deficiency. The scaling seborrhoea-like dermatosis in this patient and the glossitis in the next figure were induced in volunteers by giving the pyridoxine antagonist desoxypyridoxine. Such lesions have not been proved to occur spontaneously although it is suspected that some instances are due to pyridoxine deficiency.

111

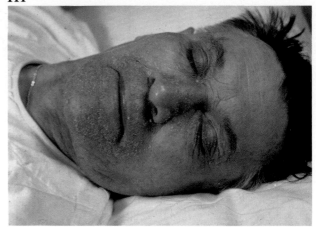

112 Glossitis in pyridoxine deficiency. This is indistinguishable from that due to deficiency of other B group vitamins (**91, 95–98, 114, 118**).

112

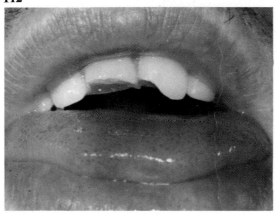

113 Ringed sideroblasts in bone marrow. These are seen in many conditions in which there is a failure in iron reutilization and hyperferraemia. Pyridoxine deficiency is only one of these. (Prussian blue, ×100)

113

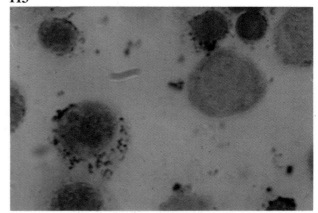

Folic acid

The daily requirement is about 400 μg. Significant losses occur in cooking and when food is not eaten fresh. Utilization is impaired in some diseases and some drugs act as antagonists. Status is usually low in pregnancy and routine supplementation is recommended.

114 The tongue in folic acid deficiency. The most marked oral manifestation is often a glossitis. The tongue becomes very red and painful and the papillae atrophy, leaving a shiny, smooth surface.

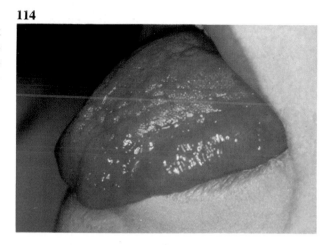
114

115 Peripheral blood in folic acid deficiency. The erythrocytes are larger than normal (macrocytosis) and consequently the mean corpuscular volume (MCV) is greater than normal, usually >96 μm^3. Many red cells are irregularly shaped (poikilocytosis). Dimorphic anaemias, in which iron deficiency is also present, may result in normalization of the red cell indices but the peripheral blood film reveals the characteristic morphology.

Polymorphonuclear leucocytes are usually reduced in number and frequently have more lobes than the normal number of 5 or 6 maximum. There is thrombocytopoenia and many platelets appear in giant form. ($\times 100$)

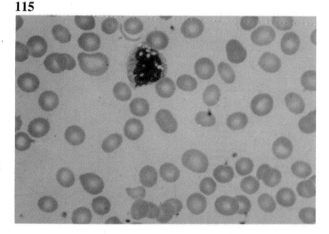
115

116 Bone marrow in folic acid deficiency. Haematopoiesis is characteristically megaloblastic. Megaloblasts are large cells with very lacy chromatin strands that have distinct parachromatin spaces between them. Mitotic figures are seen as in the upper left area here. The granulocyte nuclei have a similar appearance. The full expression of the megaloblastic appearance may be retarded by concomitant iron deficiency. The morphologic changes in peripheral blood and bone marrow are identical in deficiency of folic acid and vitamin B$_{12}$, and biochemical tests have to be relied upon for differential diagnosis ($\times 40$).

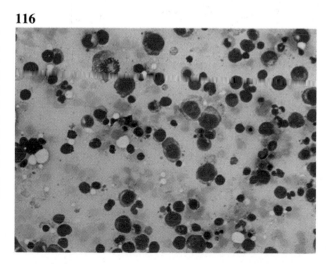
116

117 Hyperpigmentation of the skin. This patient also had a megaloblastic anaemia and recovery, including the skin, resulted from treatment with folic acid. Similar pigmentation occurs in vitamin B$_{12}$ deficiency (**120**).

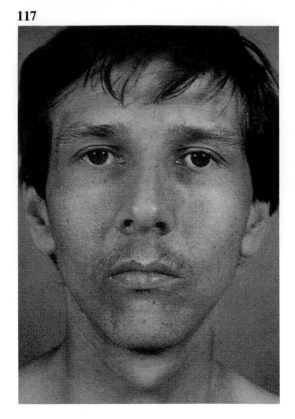

117

Vitamin B$_{12}$ (Cobalamin)

This vitamin is stored in the liver and when the dietary intake is low or absorption is impaired, as in pernicious anaemia due to absence of intrinsic factor, deficiency signs appear only after many months. The daily requirement is about 3 μg.

Vitamin B$_{12}$ occurs only in animal products and strict vegetarians (vegans) may become deficient.

Several rare forms of vitamin B$_{12}$ dependency have been described requiring massive doses (up to 100 μg daily) for their control.

118 A common initial sign in vitamin B$_{12}$ deficiency. The red sore tongue, with atrophy of the papillae is often present in pernicious anaemia and, in the case illustrated, angular stomatitis is also present.

118

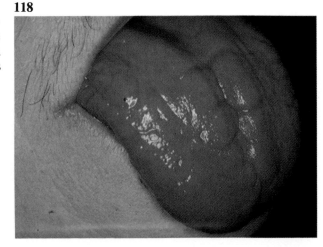

119 Pallor of pernicious anaemia. There is a pronounced lemon-yellowish tint to the skin together with faint icterus of the sclerae due to hyperbilirubinaemia. The skin is often velvety smooth, yet inelastic. It is remarkable how frequently patients have blonde or prematurely grey hair and light-coloured irides.

119

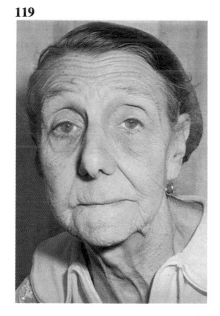

120 Hyperpigmentation of the skin. The hands of the patient should be compared with those of his normal brother. A similar change has been described in folic acid deficiency (**117**).

121 Normal pigmentation. This picture shows that after treatment with vitamin B₁₂ the hands of the patient have become the same colour as those of his brother.

120   121

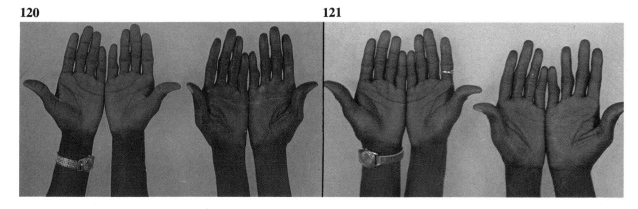

122 Subacute combined degeneration of the cord. Severe myelin degeneration affecting the posterior columns (sparing part of the cuneate tract) and lateral corticospinal tracts. Early involvement of the left anterior corticospinal tract is present. (Weigert-Pal, ×12)

122

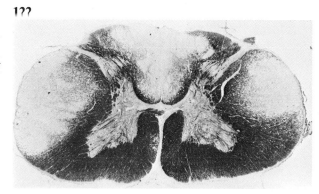

123 Nutritional retrobulbar neuropathy. Increased pallor of the temporal aspect of the optic disc is accompanied by pain behind the eyeball, photophobia and visual field defects consisting of central or centrocaecal scotomata. The papillomacular bundle of the optic nerve shows degenerative changes.

Patients are frequently deficient in vitamin B_{12} but thiamin deficiency may sometimes be responsible. Tobacco-alcohol amblyopia is generally recognized to be nutritional and not toxic in origin, but there is evidence that cyanide from pipe tobacco smoke may also play a part.

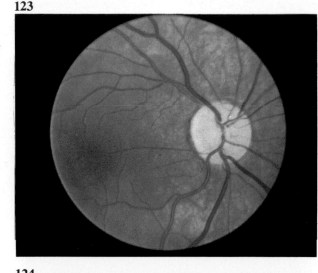

123

Biotin

124 Biotin deficiency. This rarely occurs on a natural diet but has been reported, occasionally, as in this case, in patients consuming large quantities of raw egg. This contains avidin which antagonizes the action of biotin. This patient also had cirrhosis of the liver. The skin of the hands is shiny, dry and scaly before treatment.

124

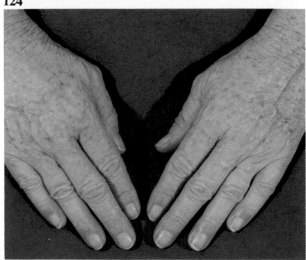

125 Biotin deficiency. The face of the same patient before treatment.

126 Biotin deficiency. The tongue of the same patient returned to normal after treatment with biotin as did the skin.

125   126

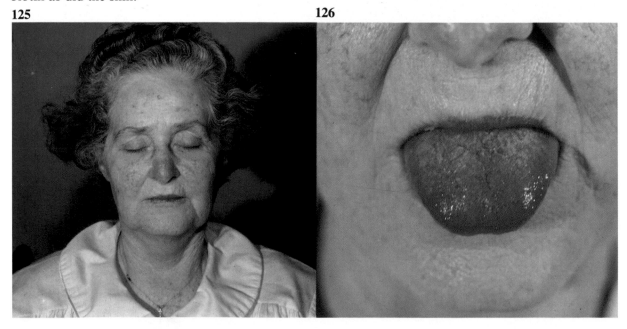

127 Biotin deficiency. The oral mucosa is reddened and sore and the tongue is a magenta colour, swollen and painful before treatment.

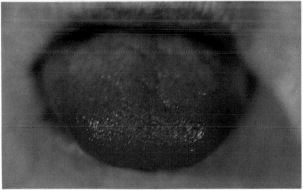

128 & 129 Biotin-dependency. A number of cases have been described in recent years of biotin-responsive disorders. Clinical features have included developmental regression and severe hypotonia, dermatitis, alopecia and defects in T-cell and B-cell immunity. Several cocarboxylase enzymes are affected and this results in increased urinary excretion of organic acids and lactic acidosis. Oral biotin, 5 mg twice daily, has proved effective.

This child shows alopecia and lack of head control before treatment. The same child at 14 months of age, after 4 months of biotin therapy, has normal posture and hair growth.

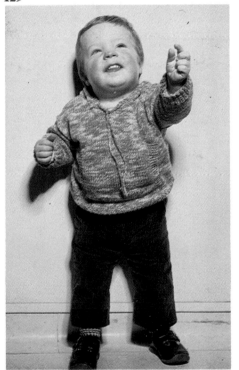

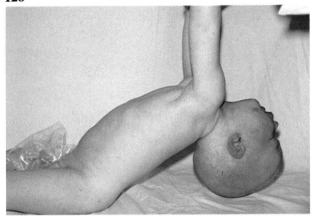

Vitamin C (Ascorbic acid)

This vitamin is abundant in citrus fruit and potatoes. It is readily destroyed by cooking. The daily requirement is generally set at 50 mg. The extremes of the life-span are particularly susceptible to deficiency. Artificially fed infants develop scurvy unless the diet is supplemented, as vitamin C is destroyed by heating the milk. Solitary old people who fail to take a balanced diet may develop gum and skin changes.

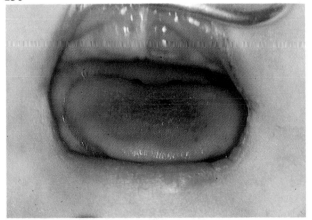

130 Gum changes in infant scurvy. The swelling and haemorrhages are confined to the areas of gum surrounding the erupting teeth.

131 Dilantoin toxicity. This should be distinguished from scorbotic gum lesions. Among the side effects of dilantoin (phenytoin sodium, diphenylhydantoin sodium) is gingival hyperplasia, occurring in about 20% on long-term therapy. It is probably the most common toxic effect in children and adolescents. The hyperplasia appears to involve altered collagen metabolism. Toothless portions of the gums are not affected. It can be minimized by good oral hygiene and does not necessitate withdrawal of medication.

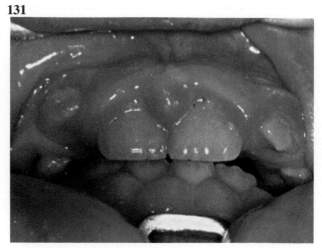

131

132 Gums in scurvy. The gums are blue-red and grossly swollen in this patient with severe scurvy. The earliest changes are swelling of the interdental papillae and tendency to bleed easily. Lesions occur only in relation to teeth and so in young infants and edentulous adults they are absent. In advanced cases there is usually an element of infection and antibiotics as well as vitamin C are required for healing.

133 Very advanced gum lesions in scurvy.

132

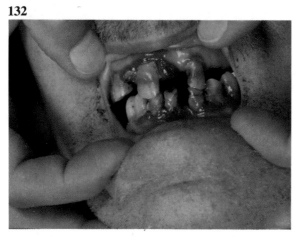

133

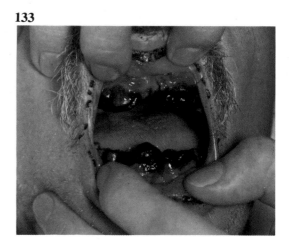

134

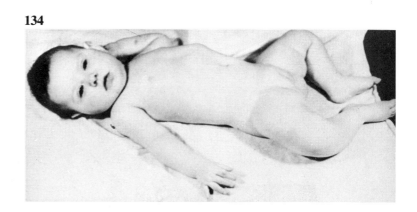

134 The 'pithed frog' position. The characteristic pseudo-paralysis of the limbs, with the legs flexed at the knees and the hips partially flexed and externally rotated, is due to the extreme pain experienced on their movement due to haemorrhages under the periosteum and sometimes infraction of an epiphysis.

135 Orbital haemorrhage. This is a dramatic but infrequent sign of scurvy. There is complete clearing with treatment.

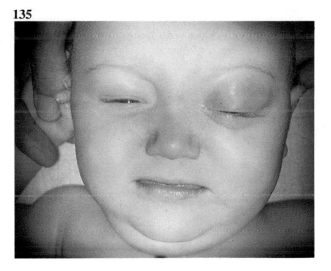

136 Splinter haemorrhages. In this unusual sign in scurvy the haemorrhages are arranged in a semi-circular lattice involving the nail beds. They are more extensive than those in sub-acute bacterial endocarditis.

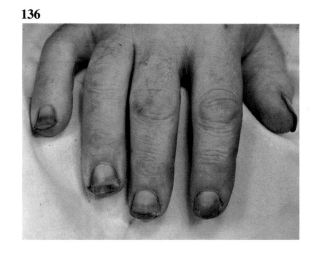

137 Perifollicular petechiae. Minimal bleeding into the hair follicles is pathognomonic of vitamin C deficiency and is often the earliest clinical manifestation. In vitamin K deficiency, thrombocytopoenia and other conditions petechiae are situated in areas of skin unrelated to the hair follicles. In perifollicular hyperkeratosis (71 & 72) there is no bleeding and hyperkeratosis is present. Ecchymoses develop in more advanced deficiency and are the most frequent sign in 'workhouse' scurvy in old men. Wound healing is markedly delayed.

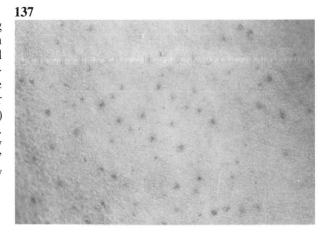

138 Bone in scurvy. Defective formation of mesenchymal tissue results from failure of deposition of inter-cellular ground substance by fibroblasts. In the shafts of long bones osteoid is not deposited by osteoblasts, the cortex is thin, trabeculae are diminished in size and haemorrhages occur under the periosteum.

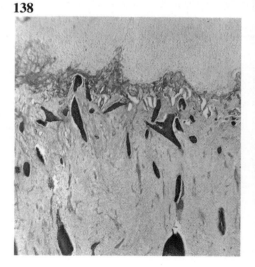

139 Bones in active scurvy. The earliest X-ray changes appear at the sites of most active bone growth; sternal end of the ribs, distal end of the femur, proximal end of the humerus, both ends of tibia and fibula, and distal ends of radius and ulna. Several characteristic signs are shown here. A zone of rarefaction immediately shaftward of the zone of provisional calcification gives rise to the 'corner fracture' sign. Atrophy of the trabecular structure and blurring of trabecular markings cause the bone to have a 'ground glass' appearance. Widening of the zone of provisional calcification causes a dense shadow at the end of the shaft (the white or Frankel's line). It also occurs at the periphery of the centres of ossification ('halo' epiphysis or 'pencilled effect').

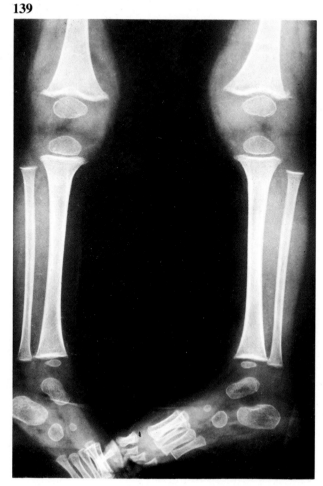

140   Bones in healing scurvy. Calcification occurring in the region of subperiosteal haemorrhage in an infant two weeks after treatment with vitamin C. The femoral epiphysis is displaced. Even the grossest deformities resolve, but radiological evidence may persist for several years.

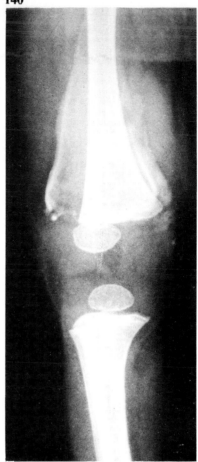

141   Active scorbutic rosary. The cartilaginous thoracic wall is pulled in by the respiratory effort.

142   Scorbutic rosary. In the healed stage in a boy who had had scurvy off and on since infancy. The sharp edges at the costochondral junctions are easily visible and this appearance is said to differentiate the scorbutic from the rachitic rosary, in which the enlarged costochondral junctions are smooth and rounded. Nevertheless, rickets and scurvy not infrequently coexist.

141

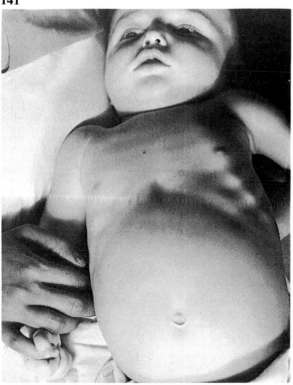

142

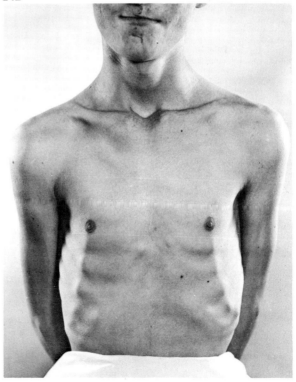

Vitamin D

The diet provides some vitamin D but most is formed from 7-dehydrocholesterol in the skin by the action of ultraviolet light. The vitamin is converted in the liver and the kidney into several metabolites that function as hormones in partici- pating in calcium and phosphorus homeostasis through their action on small intestine, bone and kidney. The recommended daily intake is $10\,\mu g$ (400 i.u.) for infants and older children and slightly less for adults.

Vitamin D deficiency

143 The skull in rickets. In infancy the frontal bones are prominent and bossed. The fontanelles are delayed in closing. The skull is soft to the touch and closely resembles pressure on a table tennis ball; the bone depresses then comes out again with exactly the same sensation. This is known as craniotabes. It is physiological at the suture lines and only indicative of rickets when it occurs also away from the suture lines.

143

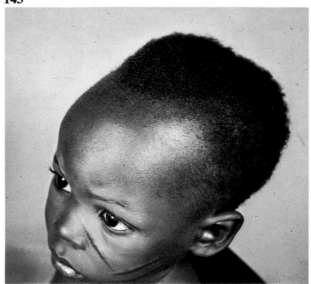

144

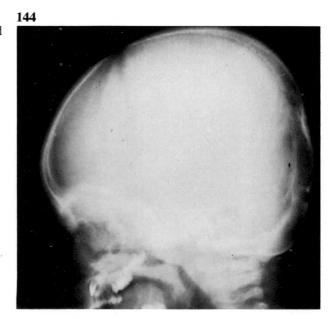

144 Skull X-ray in rickets. Frontal bossing and fontanelle separation are clearly shown.

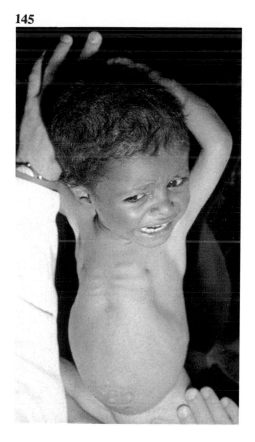

145

145 Harrison's sulcus or groove. This is a bilateral indentation of the lower ribs at the site of attachment of the diaphragm. Other deformities of the thorax, such as funnel chest, which is usually familial, and pigeon chest should not be attributed to rickets.

146 Bone in rickets. There is a failure in deposition of inorganic salts in the matrix of epiphyseal cartilage between the rows of hypertrophied cartilage cells which are not destroyed and pile up irregularly to many times their normal thickness. This gives rise to the bulky mass of intermediate zone so evident on X-ray (see **149–152**). This zone is easily compressed, deformed or displaced. There may be excessive bone destruction as the result of increased parathyroid activity and the shafts readily bend under pressure.

146

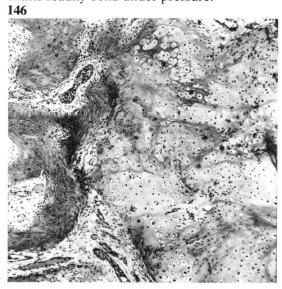

147 In the shafts there are borders of osteoid around the bone trabeculae shown here with the uncalcified osteoid stained red (Tripp and McKay stain).

147

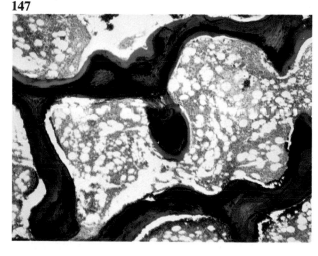

148   Bowlegs in rickets. The typical lateral curvature indicates that the weakened bones have bent after the second year as a result of standing. If severe rickets occurs before the child walks it produces a combination of bowed thighs and knock-knees. Bowing of the arms is less common, although X-ray changes at the wrist (see **149**) are almost invariably present in the infant. It precedes bowing of the legs and indicates active rickets during the last few months of the first year, when the child is crawling and pushing itself towards the erect position.

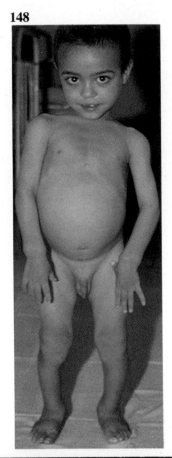

148

149   X-ray of the wrists. Some of the most characteristic and early changes take place here. The metaphyses are concave and irregular and the intervening zone of uncalcified osteoid is increased.

149

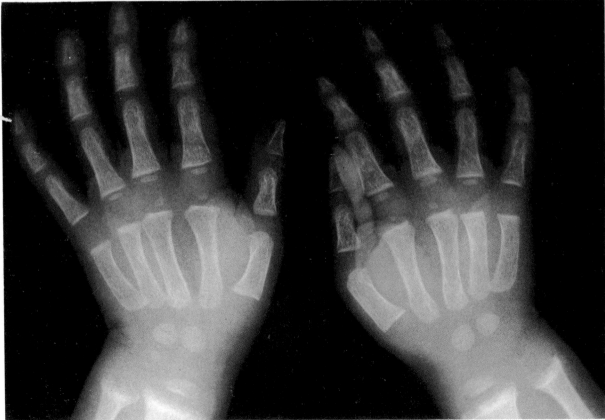

150 X-ray of the wrists. Partial healing after 4 months of treatment.

151 X-ray of the wrists. Complete healing 19 months after previous X-ray was taken.

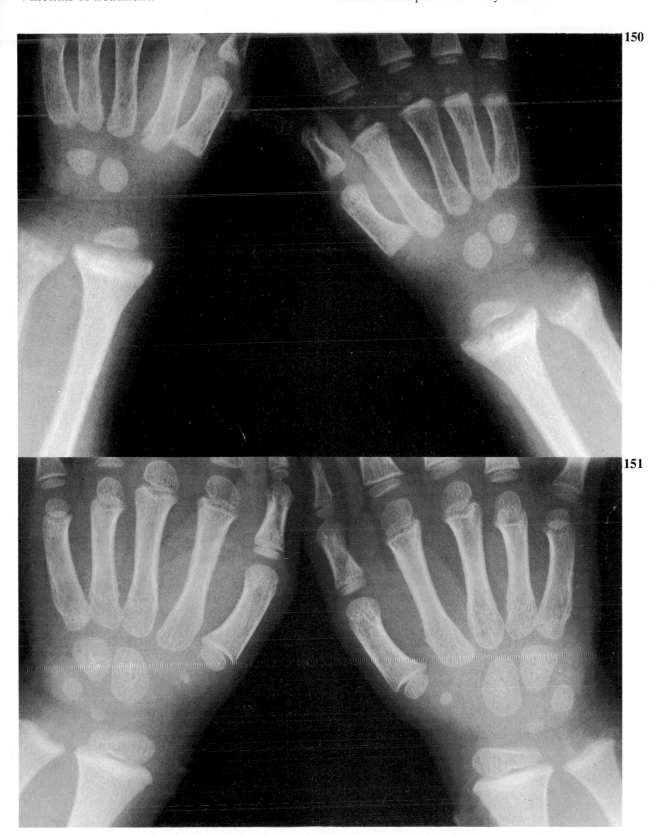

152 Active rickets of the knees. The metaphyses of the bones are concave and irregular and the zone of uncalcified osteoid is enlarged. These X-rays show the progressive changes over a 10 month period during which healing took place in this case.

152

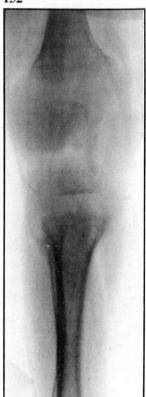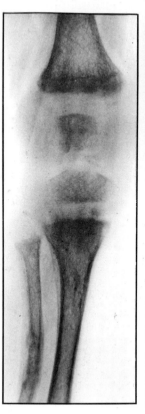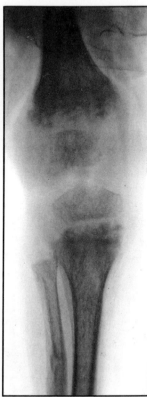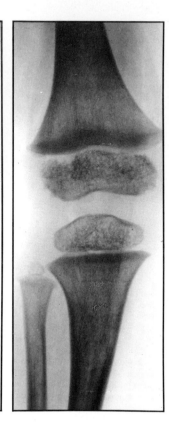

153 Excessive protective clothing. This Ethiopian mother is preventing the ultraviolet light acting on 7-dehydrocholesterol in the skin of the infant on her back to form its main source of vitamin D. Rickets is by no means uncommon in the tropics for this reason. The practice of purdah in which women in some cultures are largely confined to the house, together with their young children, has a similar result.

153

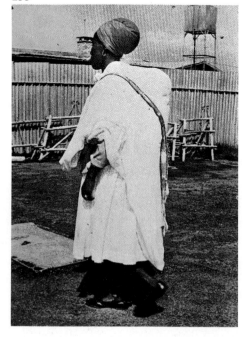

154 Vitamin D-resistant rickets. In a number of relatively rare metabolic disorders, rickets identical to that caused by a lack of vitamin D, arises from defective hydroxylation of cholecalciferol in the liver or the kidney to the active hormone form $1,25(OH)_2$ cholecalciferol. Very small daily doses of this compound or a synthetic analogue are often effective in treatment.

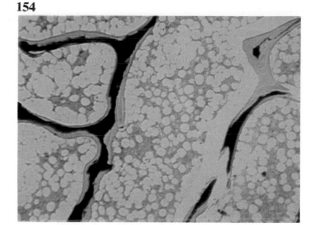

155 Osteomalacia. This is the adult form of vitamin D deficiency rickets. The section shows wide osteoid seams that cover all trabecular surfaces without increased numbers of osteoclasts.

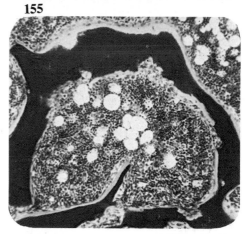

156 Looser zones (Milkman lines). These radiotranslucent zones shown here in the pelvis, and also often occurring on the axillary border of the scapula, are 'pseudofractures' (there is no bone discontinuity as in true fractures) characteristic of osteomalacia from any cause. Besides nutritional vitamin D deficiency it occurs in patients with liver or kidney disease and secondary to some drugs from interference with vitamin D hydroxylation.

Contracted pelvis due to decalicification may result in obstructed labour after a rapid succession of normal pregnancies and prolonged lactation.

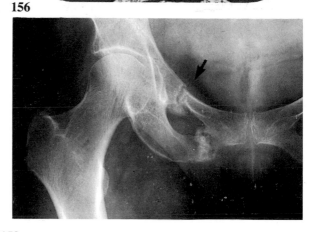

Vitamin D toxicity

157 & 158 Elfin facies of idiopathic hypercalcaemia. The characteristic facial appearance of the severe form of the disease is shown in these two patients. They are unrelated but the similarity of features might suggest a family likeness.

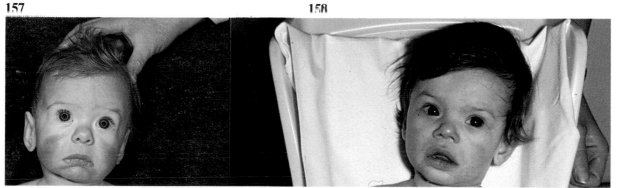

159 Idiopathic hypercalcaemia. X-ray shows increased epiphyseal bone density due to excessive calcium deposition.

159

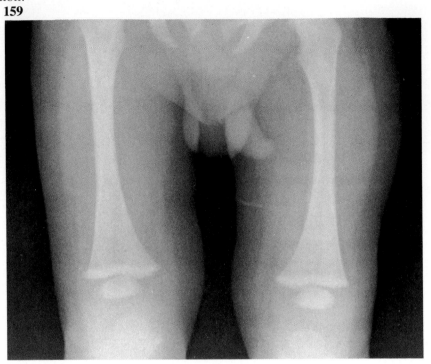

160 Idiopathic hypercalcaemia. There are marked 'growth lines' of excessive calcium deposition in this cured case.

160

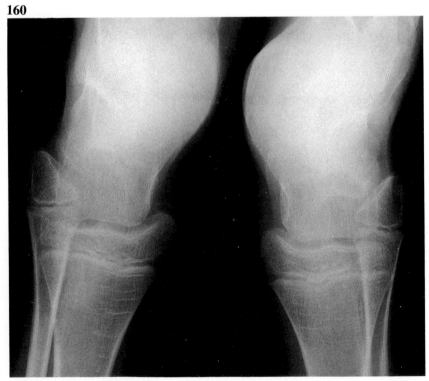

Vitamin E

The daily requirement of 10 mg of this fat-soluble vitamin is readily met by the usual adult diet. Low birth weight infants are susceptible to deficiency, especially if fed milk formulae high in poly-unsaturated fatty acids which increase vitamin E requirements. In deficiency erythrocyte haemolysis is increased and a haemolytic anaemia may develop. Fertility is impaired in animals but this has not been shown for man.

Vitamin E deficiency

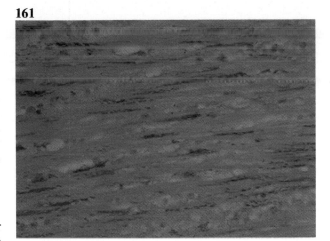

161   Brown bowel syndrome. Part of the circular layer of the tunica muscularis of the small intestine showing fusiform accumulation of lipofuscin pigment within muscle cells (Nile blue, ×200). Vitamin E deficiency is thought to play a part in this and other disorders in which there is smooth muscle myopathy probably of mitochondrial origin.

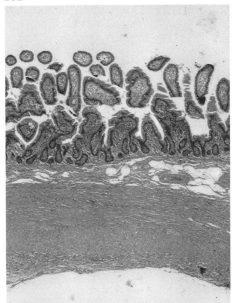

162   Brown bowel syndrome. A transverse section of the jejunum showing normal mucosa, healthy villus pattern and no evidence of mucus gland depletion. The muscularis mucosae is intact and the tunica muscularis shows no oedema or inflammation. (H&E, ×180)

Vitamin K

Vitamin K deficiency (hypoprothrombinaemia)

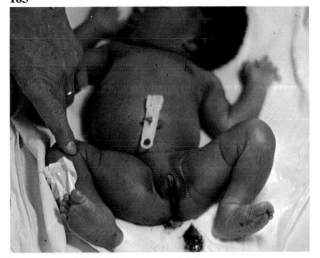

163   Haemolytic disease of the newborn. The most common sites for bleeding are the gut, producing melaena neonatorum, large cephalohaematomas, the umbilical stump, and from circumcision. Generalized ecchymoses, often without petechiae, intracranial bleeding and large intramuscular haemorrhages may develop less commonly.

Vitamin K toxicity

164 Kernicterus (bilirubin encephalopathy). Menadione and its water-soluble derivatives may cause this in low birth weight infants in relatively high doses (75 mg). It is attributed to increased haemolysis and inhibition of glucuronide formation, leading to the deposition of unconjugated bilirubin in the lipid-rich basal ganglia in the midbrain. Vitamin K is free from these effects and should be used in treatment.

The affected infant becomes lethargic, hypotonic and loses the sucking reflex. Later opisthotonos and generalized spasticity develop, followed by irregular respiration, and death results from pulmonary complications. Survivors may suffer from the post-kernicterus syndrome; high-frequency nerve deafness, athetoid cerebral palsy and dental enamel dysplasia. This patient shows neck retraction, hypertonic extensor spasm of the limbs and intense jaundice.

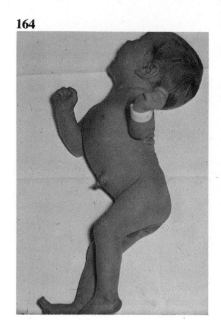

Essential fatty acids

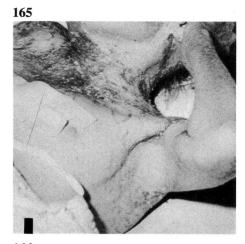

165 Essential fatty acid deficiency. Linoleic, linolenic and arachidonic acids are essential dietary constituents and in this respect resemble vitamins. They are necessary for growth, membrane formation and integrity of the skin. They are precursors of the prostaglandins.

Clinical deficiency is rare as most normal dietaries supply the body's requirements. Patients receiving fat-free parenteral nutrition have developed biochemical abnormalities and skin lesions as shown here.

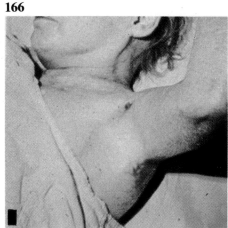

166 Essential fatty acid deficiency. Complete resolution in the same patient after 2 weeks of treatment with Intralipid.

Part 3 Element, Water and Electrolyte Deficiency and Toxicity

Iron

Only about 10% of dietary iron is absorbed and the daily requirement is 10 mg in men and 18 mg in women of the childbearing period. Iron deficiency may arise from blood loss as well as from deficient intake.

Haemochromatosis (iron overload) may be primary (idiopathic) in which a genetically determined error causes increased iron absorption from a normal diet, or secondary to increased iron intake.

Iron deficiency

167 Hypochromia and microcytosis of iron deficiency anaemia. These changes are evident only when iron deficiency is severe and they are also very nonspecific. Mean corpuscular volume (MCV) $<80\,\mu\text{m}^3$ is a sensitive index of microcytosis but is nonspecific as to cause. Early indications of iron deficiency are generally considered to be serum iron concentration $<50\,\mu\text{g/dl}$ or transferrin saturation $<15\%$ in adults. ($\times 100$)

168 Bone marrow in iron deficiency. Erythroid hypoplasia and nuclear dysplasia are present. In sections stained with Prussian blue little stainable iron will be evident. Serum ferritin is in equilibrium with storage iron in marrow, liver and other tissues and is a good early indication of iron state (normal male 94 ng/ml, normal female 34 ng/ml). ($\times 100$)

167

168

169

169 Iron deficiency anaemia. The electron microscopic appearance of the small and poorly filled erythrocytes. ($\times 8900$)

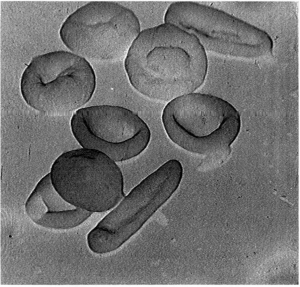

170 Koilonychia. Thinning, flattening and finally a concave or spoon-shaped appearance of the nails, as here, is typical of advanced iron deficiency. Brittle or longitudinally ridged nails are non-specific. Koilonychia is thought to be rare in young children with iron deficiency, but it was present in at least one study in a considerable proportion. The mechanism is not clear, nor is it understood why it does not occur in other forms of anaemia. It may result from prolonged exposure to soap suds and other caustic agents. When associated with fungal diseases of the skin the nails are irregularly pitted. Spoon-shaped toe nails are common in bare foot communities and are of no significance.

170

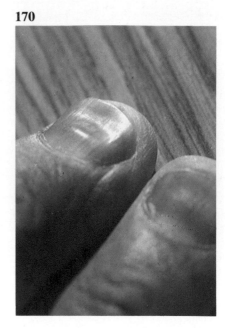

171 Skull in iron deficiency. Frontal X-ray of the skull in a young child with iron deficiency anaemia demonstrating non-uniform widening of the diploic space with a 'hair-on-end' appearance.

172 Skull in iron deficiency. Lateral view of the same patient.

171

172

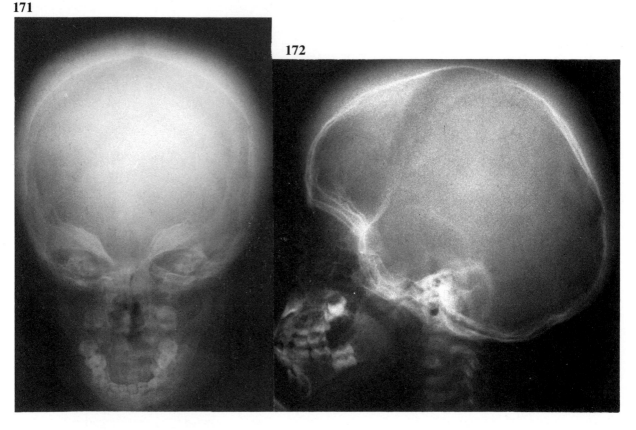

173 Plummer-Vinson (Patterson-Kelly) syndrome. There is usually a long-standing history of sidero-poenic anaemia, angular stomatitis, brittle nails (often koilonychia) and dysphagia. Six months before admission of this 71 year old woman (cases are almost always female) X-ray showed typical post-cricoid webs.

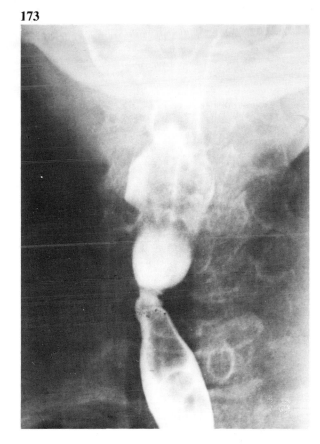

174 Plummer-Vinson syndrome. Another X-ray view of the same patient taken at the same time.

175 Plummer-Vinson syndrome. The same patient as before in whom an X-ray taken 6 months later reveals an extensive hypopharyngeal carcinoma involving both upper and lower part. The haemoglobin and serum iron were normal.

174

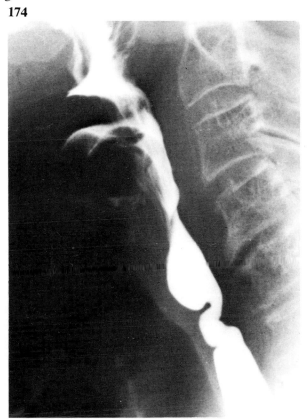

175

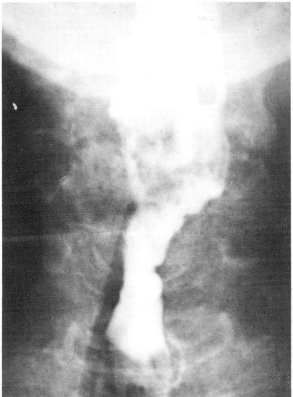

176 Plummer-Vinson syndrome. This 61 year old woman had a history of fragile nails and angular stomatitis but no known anaemia or dysphagia before onset of tumour symptoms. The X-ray shows a large exophytic carcinoma in upper part of the hypopharynx (pyriform sinus and lateral wall). Typical postcricoid Plummer-Vinson web is below the tumour region.

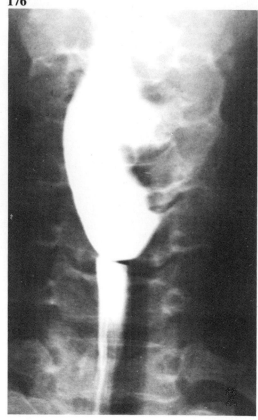

176

177 Plummer-Vinson syndrome. X-ray revealed a large postcricoid hypopharyngeal carcinoma on admission.

178 Plummer-Vinson syndrome. X-ray taken 15 months after radiation treatment revealed a typical postcricoid web shown here.

177

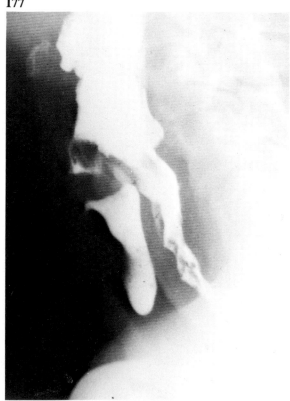

178

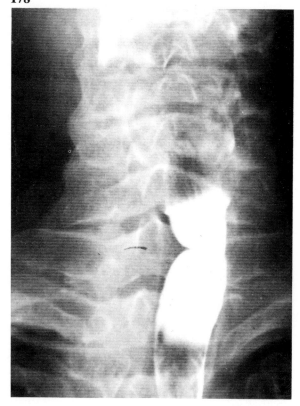

179 Plummer-Vinson syndrome. Another view of the postcricoid web in the same patient.

179

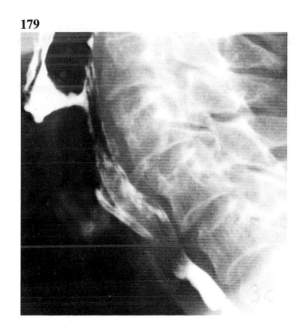

180 Plummer-Vinson syndrome. A 74 year old woman with thick leukoplakia covering a large part of the tongue and pronounced mucosal atrophy of other parts.

181 Plummer-Vinson syndrome. The same case as pictured previously. There is a slight precricoid stricture in the hypopharynx.

180

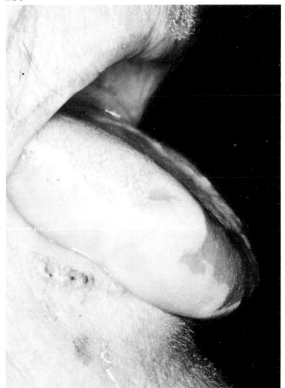

181

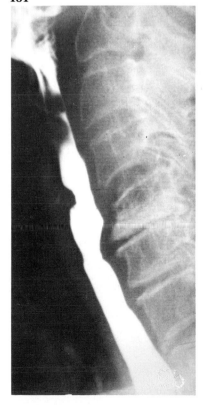

182 Plummer-Vinson syndrome. Another view of the previous case.

182

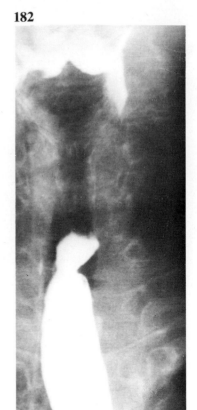

183 Plummer-Vinson syndrome. Characteristic webs are visible on X-ray in the hypopharynx. In this case a carcinoma had developed in the mouth.

184 Plummer-Vinson syndrome. Another view of the same case.

183

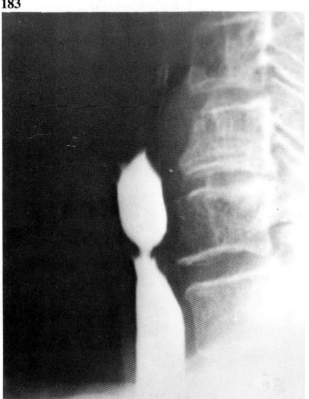

184

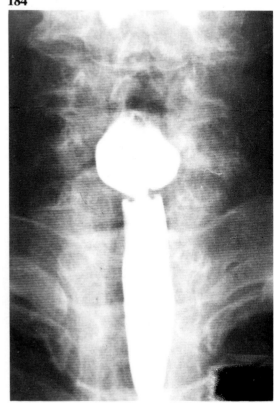

185 Plummer-Vinson syndrome. Angular stomatitis, glossitis, papillary atrophy of the tongue and
a small benign squamous cell papilloma on the
left border of the tongue are present.

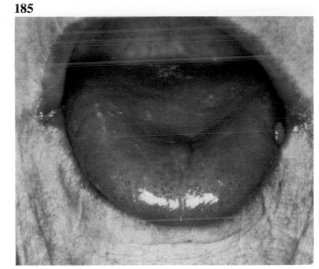

Iron toxicity

186 Haemochromatosis. The slate grey skin of
haemochromatosis (face) compared with normal
skin (hand).

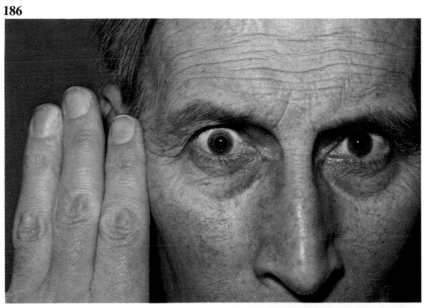

187 Bone marrow in iron overload. Prussian blue
staining reveals an excess of stainable iron, mostly
in the form of haemosiderin. (×40)

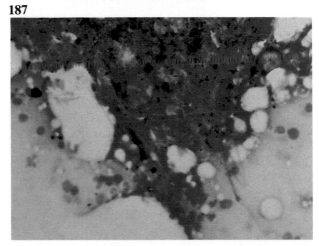

188 The liver in haemochromatosis. The liver is finely nodular, the nodules being created by finely interlacing strands of connective tissue which tend to interconnect portal triads but which also penetrate the individual lobules to separate small islands of liver substance. (H&E)

189 The liver in haemochromatosis. Large accumulations of haemosiderin occur within lymphocytes, Kupffer cells, bile duct epithelium and in the interlacing fibrous scars. The pigment is often extracellular within the scars as well as within the fibroblasts. (Prussian blue)

188

189

190 Haemochromatosis. Chondrocalcinosis in haemochromatosis, in the cartilage overlying the metacarpo-phalangeal joints of the fingers. No evidence of hyperparathyroidism, gout or pseudo gout, osteoarthritis, or Wilson's disease, all of which may be associated with calcification in cartilage.

190

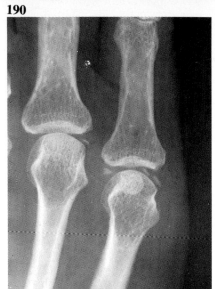

191 Haemosiderosis of the liver. Most of the iron staining is confined to the reticulo-endothelial (Kupffer) cells in the parasinusoidal spaces. It may also be localized to lungs or kidneys. The term haemosiderosis implies absence of tissue damage and when the latter occurs haemochromatosis is used (**186–190**).

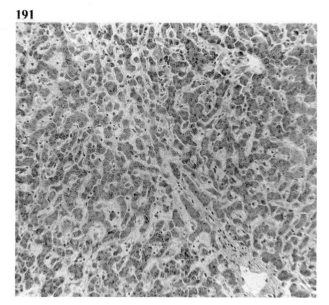

Iodine

Iodine deficiency

192 Colloid goitre, Grade 1. The thyroid gland is enlarged 4 or 5 times at this stage. Thrusting the head back makes the gland appear more prominent. A normal gland is usually described as feeling no larger than a walnut. The neck, in a relaxed position should be palpated with the fingers of both hands from behind the subject.

193 Colloid goitre, Grade 2. The goitre is easily visible with the head in the normal position.

192

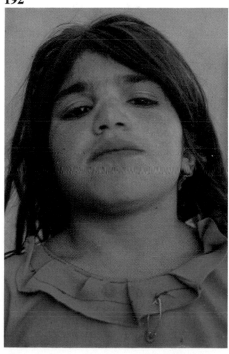

193

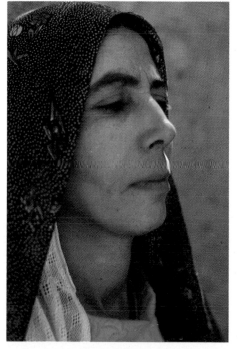

194 Colloid goitre, Grade 3. The goitre is large, visible even at a distance, disfiguring, and may cause mechanical difficulties with respiration.

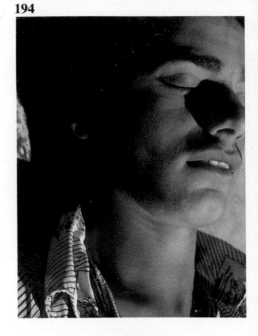

195 Cretinism in infancy. The characteristic facial appearance with protruding tongue and coarse features may not be obvious until several months after birth. Other causes of mental retardation and umbilical hernia, another feature of cretinism, must be differentiated.

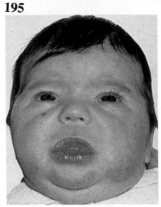

196 Cretin aged 5 years with large goitre. Mentally deficient. Several members of the family were similarly affected. They lived in an area where cretinism was endemic.

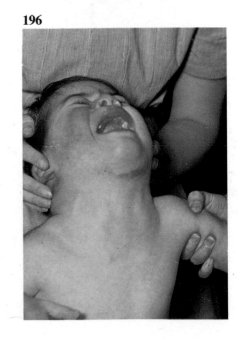

197 Endemic goitre and cretinism in Bolivia. The mother, on the left, is goitrous but otherwise normal. The daughter is goitrous, mentally retarded, and a deaf mute, but of normal stature and clinically euthyroid.

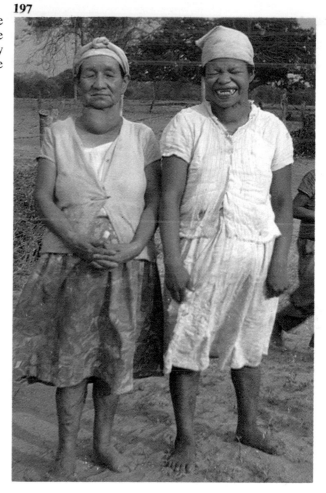

198 Colloid goitre. The follicles are distended with colloid and the epithelial lining is flattened. There is a scant amount of interacinar connective tissue devoid of significant lymphoid infiltrate. Vascularization is diminished.

199 Colloid goitre. The thyroid gland is considerably enlarged and follicles of varying size can be seen distended with colloid.

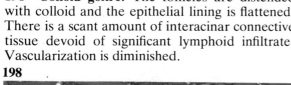

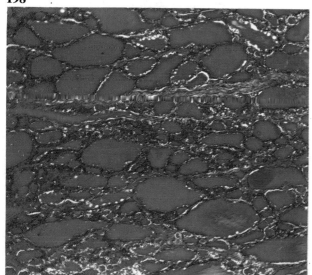

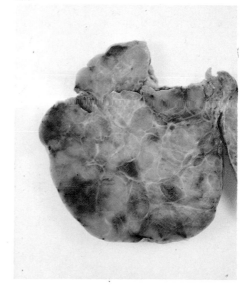

200 Toxic goitre. This is not due to iodine deficiency. There are signs of increased metabolism. This is hyperthyroidism (Grave's disease, exophthalmic goitre, thyrotoxicosis).

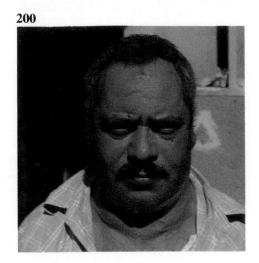

Fluorine

Fluorine deficiency

201 Dental caries. This is a localized progressive loss of tooth substance initiated by demineralization of the tooth surface by organic acids. These are produced by enzymes of cariogenic bacteria (especially *streptococcus mutans*) that ferment sugars trapped in the tooth-adherent bacterial film called dental plaque. Oral hygiene is clearly of paramount importance in prevention but fluoride ions have been shown to inhibit caries by replacing some of the hydroxyl ions in tooth hydroxyapatite to form a relatively acid-insoluble fluorhydroxyapatite.

Added fluoride is ineffective against fissure caries that affects the surfaces of the teeth in the 6 to 12 year old age group but does prevent caries that tends to attack the adjacent base areas of teeth in young adults.

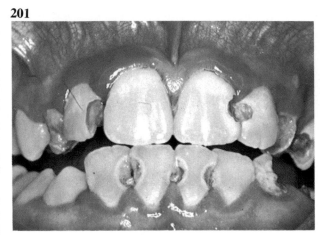

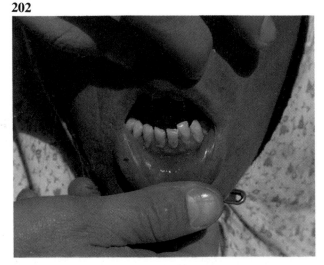

202 Pyorrhoea or periodontitis. There is an inflammatory breakdown of the supporting structures of the roots (gingiva and periodontal ligament) with a resultant loss of alveolar bone. The gums are hyperaemic and bleed easily but there is no hypertrophy. Although common in undernourished subjects there is no evidence that nutritional deficiency plays a part, and it must be distinguished from scurvy (**132 & 133**).

Fluorine toxicity

203 Mottled enamel in fluorosis. The affected areas are 'paper-white', yellowish or brownish and are usually situated on or near the tips of cusps or incisal edges. They shade off imperceptibly into the surrounding normal enamel. Fluorosis is most frequent on teeth that calcify slowly (cuspids, bicuspids, second and third molars) and is less marked on lower than upper incisors. Usually seen on six or eight homologous teeth, it is extremely rare on deciduous teeth. This degree of discolouration usually follows several years of constant exposure to concentrations up to about 10 times the normal (about 1 part per million) of fluorine in the drinking water. The teeth of most inhabitants of such an area are affected by school age. There is no damage to teeth at this stage.

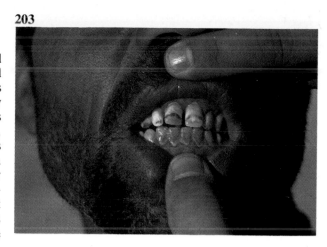

204 Enamel hypoplasia. The central part of the upper incisors is usually affected as in this case. It is not known to be related to nutritional deficiency. It can be distinguished from the mottling of fluorosis by the pigmentation being present at the time of eruption and by the etched and roughened surface of the enamel.

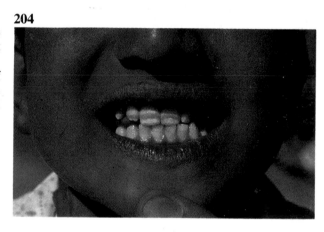

205 Pitting and mottling of the teeth. In prolonged and extreme fluorosis the weakened enamel is lost, resulting in pits. As in the earlier stage of mottling alone the upper incisors are more severely affected with the confluence of isolated pits into bands of erosion. In parts of India, the Arabian Gulf and Africa lifelong consumption of drinking water with many times the normal concentration of fluorine results in skeletal fluorosis. Marked osteosclerosis of the spine causes severe pain and limitation of movement and marked genu valgum also occurs.

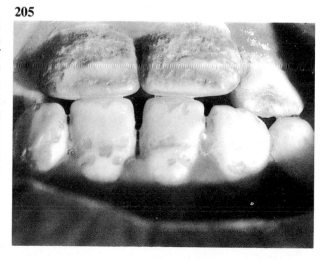

Water and electrolytes

206 Overhydration. Girl of 2 months, weight 5500 g (75th centile for 4 months). Birthweight was 3200 g. The feeding formula contained excess of carbohydrates and lack of protein, leading to increased fluid retention and apparent plumpness easily lost during recurrent illness.

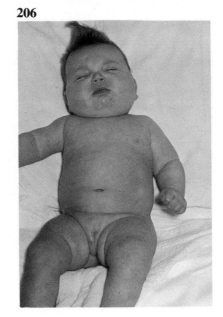

207 Hypernatraemia. Section through the cerebellum in a fatal case of salt poisoning showing a subarachnoid haemorrhage, vascular dilation and congestion and a small cortical haemorrhage. (Pickworth-Lepehne stain, ×50)

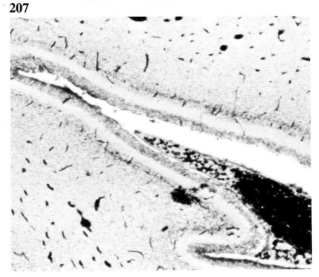

208 Hypernatraemia. Section through the cerebral cortex and subcortical white matter showing widespread capillary and venous congestion with red blood cell diapedesis and small haemorrhages. (Pickworth-Lepehne stain, ×50)

209 Hypernatraemia. Section of the kidney of an infant dying after 3 days from salt poisoning, showing extensive sub-basilar vacuolation in renal tubules at all levels of the nephron. Note that the cytoplasm may be lifted off the basement membrane and the lumen obliterated.

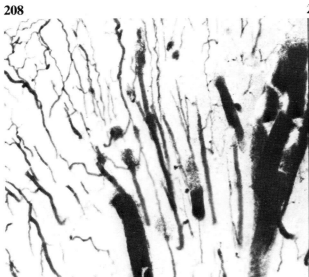

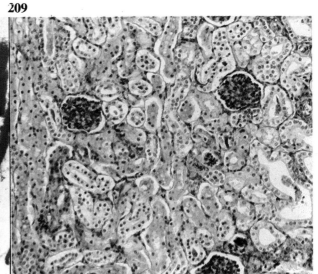

Calcium

Deficiency and excess do not arise from dietary imbalance alone. Both are frequently associated with disorders of vitamin D metabolism (143–160). One condition of excessive calcium deposition unrelated to vitamin D that responds to a reduced calcium intake is osteopetrosis.

Calcium excess

210 & 211   Osteopetrosis or marble bone disease. A severe recessive form of this uncommon condition often leads to death in infancy. A milder dominant form is diagnosed in later childhood or adolescence. X-ray of the wrists, hands and pelvic region reveals marked density of bone and lack of moulding. Treatment consists of a low calcium diet combined with corticosteroids and splenectomy.

210

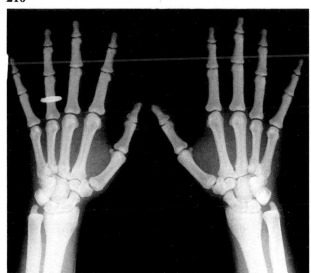

211

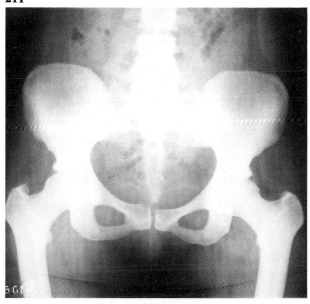

Zinc

212 Acrodermatitis enteropathica. This is an inherited, previously fatal, disorder characterized by a psoriasiform dermatitis, often affecting the whole body, diarrhoea, hair loss, paronychia and growth retardation. It is due to a defect in the absorption of zinc and responds dramatically to this trace element.

A syndrome of growth retardation and hypogonadism responding to zinc has been described in the Middle East. Low zinc status may occur in many diseases and is probably sometimes responsible for failure to thrive and hypogeusia (impaired taste) in children, and night blindness in adults with liver disease or malabsorption.

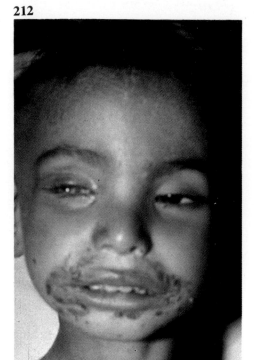

Copper

This trace element is widely distributed in foodstuffs and the daily requirement of about 2 mg is readily provided. Undernourished infants fed on a mainly milk diet have developed an anaemia that responds to copper administration. Menke's kinky hair syndrome (**219**) is due to a defect in copper absorption.

Copper toxicity occurs in Wilson's disease, with low circulating caeruloplasmin levels and damage due to deposition of copper in tissue, notably in brain, liver, eye and kidney. Foods rich in copper should be avoided, and pyridoxine assists the action of penicillamine in chelating copper from tissues.

Evidence has recently been provided that infantile biliary cirrhosis is due to a defect in copper metabolism.

Copper excess

213 Hepato-lenticular degeneration (Wilson's disease). Right cerebral hemisphere in coronal section to show shrinkage of the putamen and globus pallidus. (×1.6)

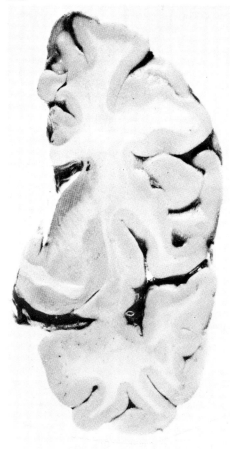

214 Hepato-lenticular degeneration (Wilson's disease). The trapezoid body of the pons shows microcystic degeneration, astrocytic hyperplasia and several Opalski cells, which have pink granular cytoplasm and characteristically small round or ovoid nucleus. (H&E, ×160)

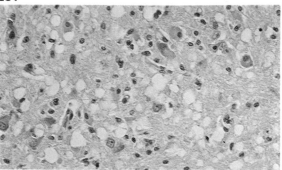
214

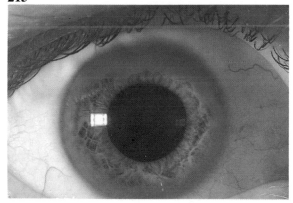
215

215 Cornea in Wilson's disease. Copper deposits in Descemet's membrane in the corneal periphery produce the pathognomonic Kayser-Fleischer ring. This is a complete or incomplete brown to green ring near the limbus, most noticeable superiorly and inferiorly, best seen in the early stages with the gonioprism.

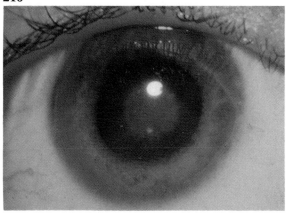
216

216 The lens in Wilson's disease. Copper deposition is present, resulting in the characteristic 'sun flower' cataract.

217 The lens in Wilson's disease. A painting (by Mr T.R. Tarrant) of the same eye as in the previous figure, of the anterior and posterior surfaces of the lens and the optical section of the lens (arrowed).

218 The lens in Wilson's disease. The lens has been photographed as in **216** after 5 years of treatment with penicillamine. There is total clearing of the copper deposits.

217
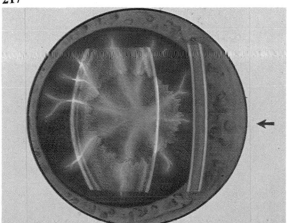

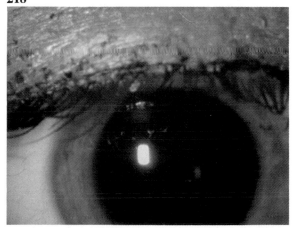
218

Copper deficiency

219 Menke's kinky hair syndrome. The typical appearance of the face and sparse and brittle hair in this sex-linked disorder caused by a defect in intestinal copper absorption. There is also retarded growth, progressive cerebral degeneration, arterial lesions and scurvy-like bone changes. Early treatment with copper salts intravenously daily may alleviate the condition.

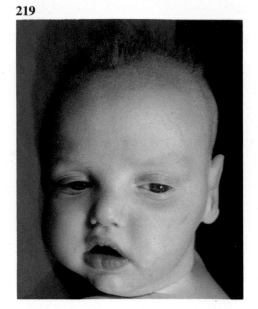

Cobalt

220 Cobalt toxicity. Fatal poisoning with cobalt has been reported as a result of drinking contaminated beer, industrial exposure and in patients on maintenance haemodialysis either with or without cobalt therapy.

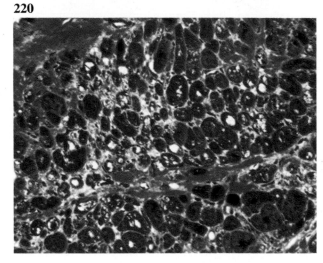

221 Cobalt cardiomyopathy. These sections show the characteristic areas of myocardial necrosis, with vacuolated fibres that have lost their striations, and irregular, very large nuclei. Neutron activation analysis for cobalt showed about 40 times the normal concentration.

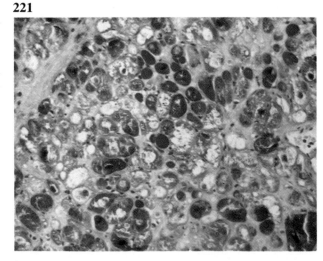

222 Cobalt toxicity. X-ray of the chest on admission showing the grossly dilated heart.

222

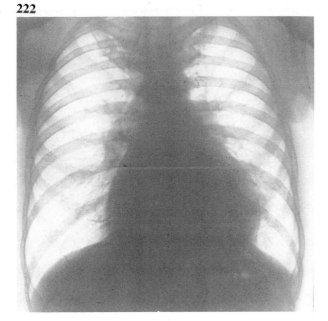

223 Cobalt toxicity. The same patient 4 months after discharge showing the return of the heart to normal size.

223

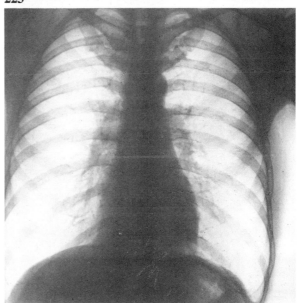

224 Cobalt toxicity. Electrocardiogram taken on admission showing prominent P waves and low voltage in the upper tracing.

224

225 Cobalt toxicity. The record of the same patient 9 months later showing considerable improvement.

225

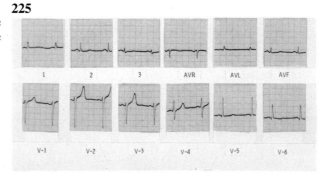

Part 4   Diet-Responsive Metabolic Disorders

The large number of metabolic disorders is constantly being added to. Many of these are extremely rare while some of them are major contributors to human morbidity and mortality. For the most part they are inherited diseases involving disorders of lipid, carbohydrate or amino acid metabolism. While none of them is directly attributable to nutritional deficiency nutrition is invariably involved to a greater or lesser extent.

Some of the most important among these conditions respond completely or in part to dietary measures and these have been included here. For a number this is the only form of treatment available.

Obesity

The reasons why a high proportion of individuals tend to accumulate excessive amounts of adipose tissue are not fully understood. Heredity, culture and activity are as important as overeating. The importance of overfeeding in infancy in predisposing to adult obesity has not been conclusively demonstrated. Fashion in slimming diets constantly changes and only serves to emphasize that there is no short cut to weight loss and that this can only be achieved by a life-long restriction of total energy intake to balance energy expenditure.

226

226   Obese girl and normal child of the same age. Weight difference was 15.25 kg. Note the difference in height.

227   Obesity, adipose dimpling and oedema. No pitting. There may be oedema as a secondary effect due to the sheer physical weight obstructing the venous and lymphatic return, as can be seen in the feet. This oedema will pit.

227

228   Obesity. The roundness and fatness of the face in obesity must be differentiated from the appearance of hyperadrenocorticolism. In the latter there is oedema of the facial tissues and frequently erythema.

228

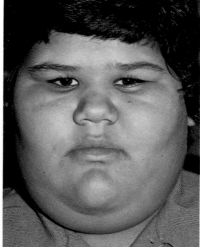

229 Calorie excess. Girl of 4 months, weight 9070 g (75th centile for 9 months). Birth weight was 3850 g. Overfeeding was the only cause of the excess deposition of adipose tissue on the face, buttocks and limbs, and the Cushingoid appearance.

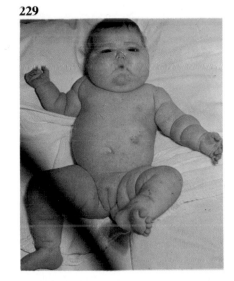

229

230 Precocious development. Girl aged 10 years. Weight 65 kg, height 165 cm corresponding to the 75th centile for 15 years. The distribution of fat tissue on the breasts and abdomen with relatively slim limbs is of adult type. The girl was a compulsive eater (hyperphagia).

230

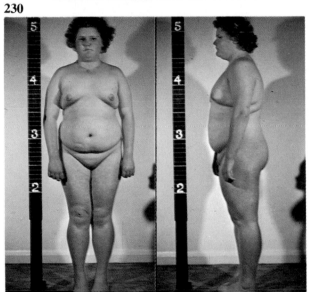

231 Postural defects in obesity. The 3 year old boy shows valgus deformity of the legs, and lordosis, which may persist throughout life.

231

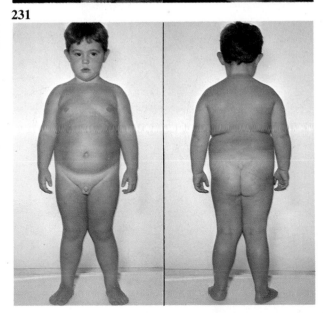

232 Obesity. The centimetre scale indicates the extent to which adipose tissue may accumulate subcutaneously.

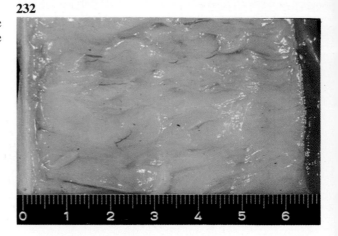

Disorders of lipid metabolism

Hyperlipoproteinaemias

This complex group of disorders of lipid metabolism may be *acquired* in association with many diseases, for example diabetes mellitus, thyroid and liver diseases, or *familial*. The latter are classified according to the scheme proposed by Fredrickson. Type I (familial lipoprotein lipase deficiency) responds to a very low fat diet. Type II (a and b) (familial hypercholesterolaemia) is partially responsive to limitation of dietary cholesterol and saturated fat. Diet is most effective in Type III in which carbohydrate is restricted and much of the fat is in the form of polyunsaturated fatty acids. Type IV usually responds to weight reduction and carbohydrate restriction, and Type V to strict energy balance and limitation of dietary fat.

233 Tendon xanthomata. These consist of lipid accumulation of tissues in association with large foam cells. Type IIa, familial hyperbetalipoproteinaemia or hypercholesterolaemia is usually present. In a rare familial condition with normal lipoproteins the upper part of the Achilles tendon is affected, followed by pulmonary insufficiency, dementia and spastic ataxia due to deposits of cholestoral and cholestanol. The metabolic defect has not been established.

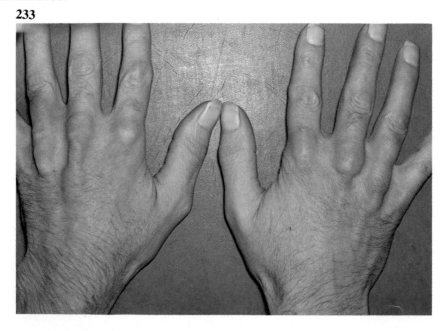

234 Cutaneous xanthomata (xanthoma tuberosum). Besides the elbows, the buttocks, palms and viscera are often affected. Type IIa, and less commonly Types IIb or III hyperlipoproteinaemia accompanies these lesions. In juveniles the plasma lipids may be normal.

234

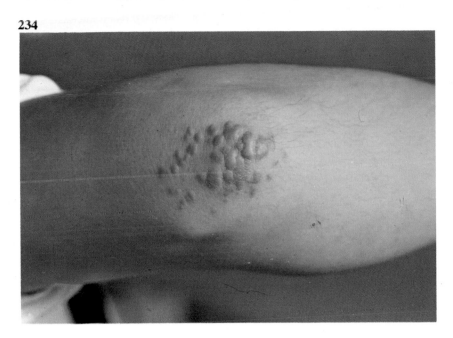

235 Xanthelasma (xanthoma planum). The lesions usually appear in the 3rd or 4th decades and develop symmetrically on the inner third of the upper lids and may also involve the lower lids. They are less frequently associated with hyperbetalipoproteinaemia than xanthomata elsewhere.

235

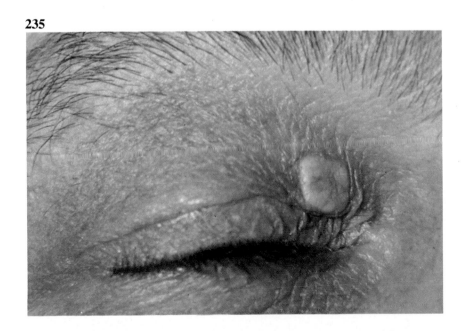

236 Corneal arcus. This is an infiltration of lipid forming a complete ring in the paralimbal periphery of the cornea. In young and middle aged subjects hyperlipoproteinaemia is often present, together with xanthoma or xanthelasma, and the term premature arcus and not arcus senilis should be used.

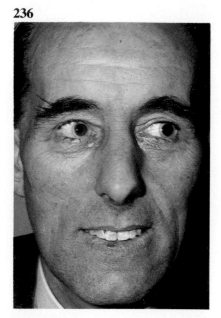

237 Arcus senilis (gerontoxon). In old age the plasma lipids are usually normal and other signs of disturbed lipid metabolism are absent.

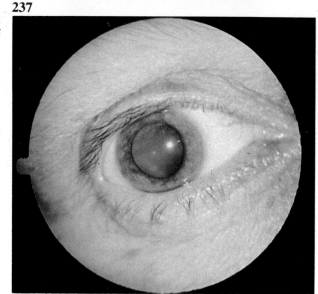

Atherosclerosis

Lipid deposition in and hardening of the arteries constitute atherosclerosis, and this with subsequent thrombus formation in coronary and cerebral vessels is the process underlying most instances of heart attacks and strokes. Among the many factors associated with atherosclerosis the composition of the diet holds a prominent place. There is still considerable controversy concerning the importance of diets high in sugar or cholesterol, or low in fibre or polyunsaturated fatty acids. It is generally accepted that atherosclerosis and its complications are most prevalent in communities consuming a diet high in saturated fat.

238 Atheromatous aortic aneurysm. There is gross atheromatous plaque formation, and weakening of the wall has resulted in aneurysm formation.

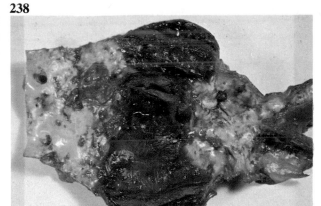

238

239 Coronary artery thrombosis. Fatty streaks evolve into raised subintimal plaques which encroach on the vascular lumen. Superimposed thrombosis occurs on fissured, or more often ulcerated lesions, as here.

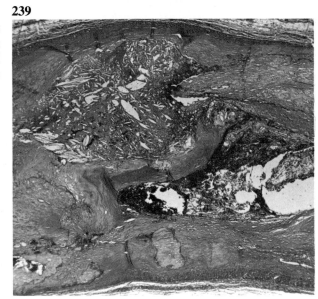

239

Cholelithiasis

Dietary management cannot influence the process of gall stone formation. Fried fat does tend to precipitate attacks of acute cholecystitis. As the stones are composed largely of cholesterol the dietary intake should be restricted. This measure has also been shown to enhance the effect of chenic acid in dissolving the stones.

240 Cholelithiasis. A cholesterol stone is shown, against a centimetre scale, and chronic cholecystitis is present.

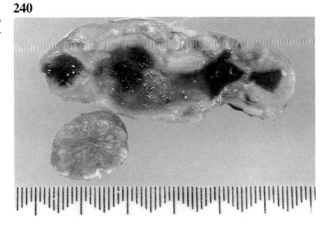

240

Abetalipoproteinaemia

This autosomal recessive disorder is also known as the Bassen-Kornzweig syndrome. Malabsorption, posterior column disease, misshapen erythrocytes called acanthocytes and cardiovascular disease are common clinical features. Besides the retinal degeneration pictured here other eye changes include nystagmus, strabismus, ptosis and colour vision defects. Transport of fat and fat-soluble vitamins is impaired. A low fat diet controls the malabsorption and promotes catch-up growth. Supplementation with vitamins A and E has been claimed to improve the retinal changes.

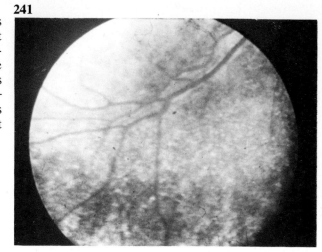

241 **Retina in abetalipoproteinaemia.** There is retinal pigmentary degeneration without evident narrowing and pigment clumping in the mid-periphery. Some patients present a picture resembling retinitis punctata albescens, as does this one. Optic nerve pallor and posterior degeneration may occur. Nystagmus, strabismus and ptosis are common. A blue-yellow colour vision defect may be detected. Night blindness is common.

Refsum's disease

This recessively inherited disorder is due to the absence of phytanic acid hydroxylase which causes the accumulation of phytanic acid in tissues. Clinical features besides those pictured here include cerebellar ataxia, peripheral polyneuropathy, tremors, paresis and sensory loss. Heart disease, deafness and ichthyosis also occur.

Dietary management is designed to avoid foods rich in phytanic acid such as fat meat and fish, whole dairy products, most vegetables and nuts.

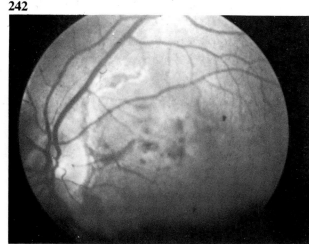

242 **Retina in Refsum's disease.** Night blindness is often the earliest abnormality. The electroretinogram (ERG) may be diminished or extinct. Visual field loss is common. Posterior cortical or subcapsular cataracts are present in about 35% of cases. This case shows pallor of the optic nerve head, arteriolar narrowing and retinal pigmentary disturbance.

243 Retina in Refsum's disease. The peripheral retina shows mottling, 'salt and pepper' pattern, and 'bone spicule' pigmentary degeneration.

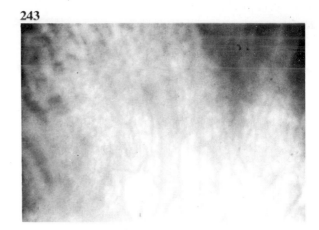

243

Disorders of carbohydrate metabolism
Diabetes mellitus

This common and complex group of disorders involving genetic predisposition and impaired secretion of insulin by the pancreas has effects on most organs of the body. Only the two most common and serious ocular manifestations are illustrated here.

Dietary measures are of special importance in maturity-onset diabetics. They are often overweight and correction of this alone may be all that is required. It has long been the practice to restrict carbohydrate intake and this inevitably means a high fat diet if energy requirements are to be met. The common association of diabetes with atherosclerosis (**238 & 239**) may be partly attributable to a diet high in saturated fat. Present practice is not to limit carbohydrate intake (providing about 60% of energy needs) and for fat to contribute about 30% with a ratio of polyunsaturated fat: other fat greater than 1:1.

244 Diabetic cataract. The most common type of true diabetic cataract, shown here, consists of posterior subcapsular opacity with radial striae extending into it from the equatorial zone. Less frequently numerous white flaky opacities in the cortex give a snowstorm appearance. In more advanced cases lens fibres become distorted with intervening vacuoles.

'Senile' cataract, distinguished by the uniform opacification, occurs more frequently and at an earlier age in diabetics.

245 Diabetic retinopathy. Note the vascular changes, predominantly at the posterior pole of the eye, with 'dot and blot' haemorrhages and hard exudates arranged side by side. There are minimal arterio-venous changes. Microaneurysms are a characteristic feature.

Iridopathy leading to glaucoma and vitreous haemorrhages also occur.

244

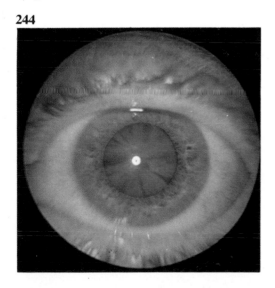

245

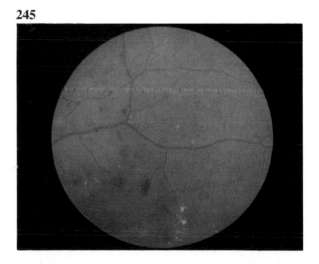

Glycogen storage diseases

There are eight types of these rare enzyme disorders of glycogen metabolism; in only Types I and III of which is dietary management effective. Type I is glucose-6-phosphatase deficiency or Von Gierke's disease. Sugars other than glucose should be avoided. Type III or debrancher enzyme deficiency results in milder degrees of growth failure and hepatomegaly than Type I. In this type a high protein diet is indicated.

246 **Glycogen storage disease.** This picture shows hepatomegaly and stunting in a patient with Type III at 7 years of age.

247 This is the same patient at 17 years of age; growth and development are normal, the liver is not enlarged and there are no symptoms.

246   **247**

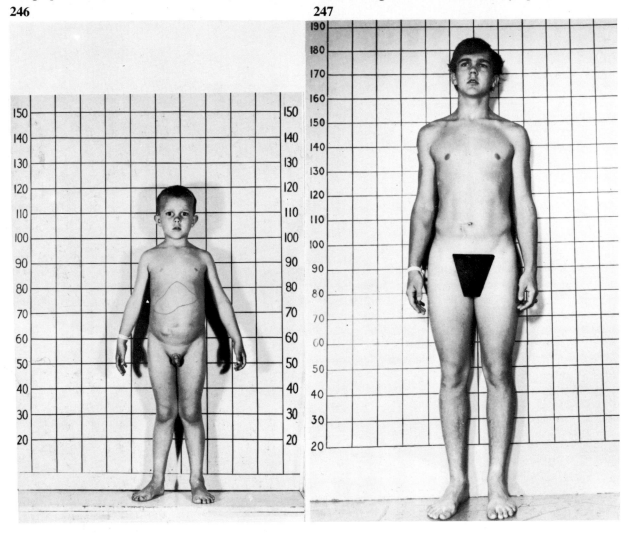

Galactosaemia

This disorder results from absence of the enzyme galactose-1-phosphate uridyltransferase. Galactose is part of the molecule of lactose, milk sugar, and accumulates in the tissues. There is growth failure and mental retardation.

Proprietary galactose-free milk instituted early permits normal development. Galactokinase deficiency, also causing cataract, is a much rarer disorder and responds similarly to treatment.

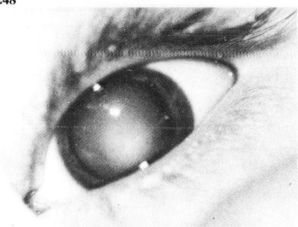

248 Galactosaemia. The first evidence may be cataract as in this infant.

249 Liver in galactosaemia. Biopsy specimen from an infant showing pseudoacinus and fatty change in the parenchymal cells. (H&E, ×500)

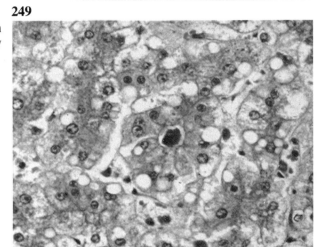

Disorders of amino acid metabolism

250 Phenylketonuria. This is one of the more common and most studied aminoacidopathies. Several forms have been described but most commonly there is deficiency of liver phenylalanine hydroxylase. Mental retardation is severe in the untreated case. A diet providing not more than between 200 and 500 mg phenylalanine per day needs to be given at least for the first 6 years of life and probably longer to ensure full growth and development. Over restriction results in protein deficiency.

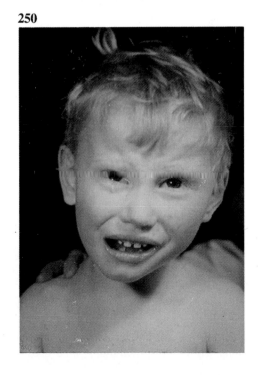

251 Maple syrup urine disease. This is one of a number of disorders involving metabolism of the branched-chain keto amino acids. Within a few days of birth feeding difficulties, hypertonicity and a shrill cry develop and unless these amino acids are restricted in the diet neurological damage and death will follow. This photomicrograph shows spongy degenerative changes in the globus pallidus.

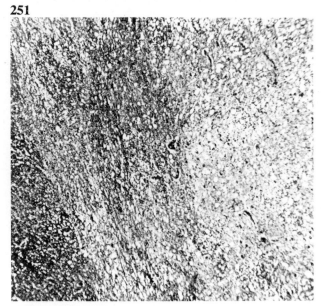

252 Hartnup disease. This appearance resembling Casal's necklace should suggest the possibility of Hartnup disease. In this aminoacidopathy there is an absorption defect of tryptophan. There is a dermatosis identical to that of pellagra, temporary cerebellar ataxia and a constant aminoaciduria. Nicotinamide about 100 mg daily results in cure.

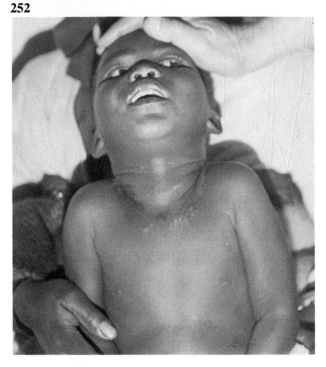

253 Tyrosinaemia (tyrosinosis). Bilateral corneal ulceration is common, together with liver and renal tubular dysfunction. A diet low in phenylalanine and tyrosine may permit normal growth and development.

253

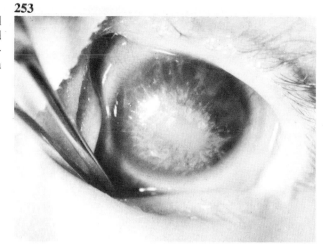

254

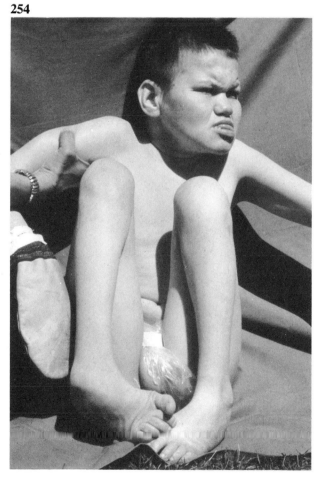

254 Hyperlysinaemia. This rare disorder of lysine metabolism may result in severe mental retardation and a variety of other clinical features. A diet low in lysine as soon as the diagnosis is made is advocated.

255 Homocystinuria. Cystothionine ß-synthase that facilitates the condensation of homocystine with serine to yield cystathionine is lacking. Skeletal damage is prominent. A low protein, low methionine diet is advocated and some patients respond to large doses of vitamin B₆. The first X-ray of an 18 year old girl shows osteoporosis and characteristic biconcavity or 'cod fish' deformity of the vertebrae, seen more markedly in the second X-ray of an 11 year old girl.

255

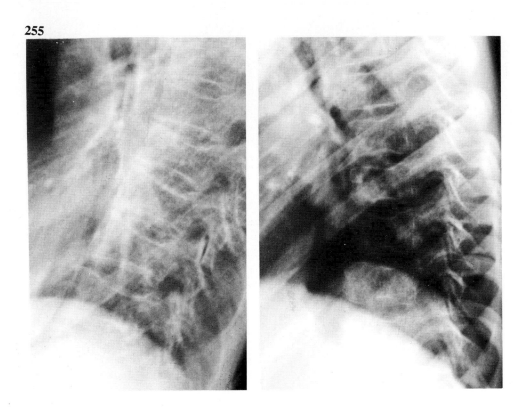

256 Homocystinuria. X-ray of the lower femur and knee shows osteoporosis and widening of the distal metaphysis and epiphysis of the femur.

256

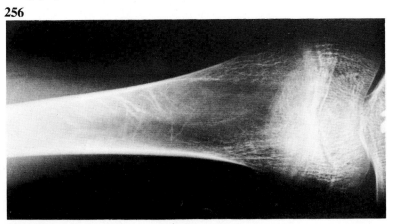

257 Cystinosis. Cystine is deposited in many tissues, shown here in the cornea, and especially as urinary calculi, in this relatively common autosomal recessive disorder. The diet should be relatively low in protein and methionine, but a high fluid intake and alkalinization of the urine are the most important measures.

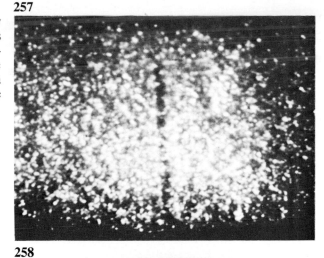

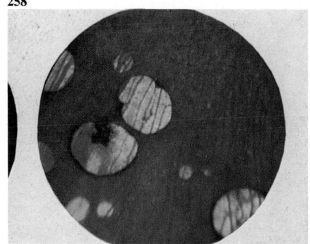

258 Hyperornithinaemia. Ornithine transaminase is deficient in this rare disorder, and gyrate atrophy of the retina, shown here, is characteristic. Hyperammonaemia occurs, as it does in many disorders affecting urea cycle enzymes, with vomiting, somnolence and convulsions leading to coma and death, or mental retardation and neurological disorders in survivors. Treatment is difficult but dietary protein should be restricted to a minimum necessary to meet amino acid requirements.

Gout

This disorder results, in those with a genetic predisposition, from biochemical abnormalities causing excessive uric acid formation and diminished renal excretion. Drug treatment controls blood uric acid and relieves acute inflammation of the affected joints.

The diet should be low in purines. Meat intake should be restricted and rich sources such as liver, kidney, sweatbread, brain, fish roe, sardine, crab, anchovy, sprats, peas and beans should be avoided.

259 Gouty tophus. This comprises a mass of urate crystals in the affected joint, surrounded by an inflammatory response composed of young fibroblasts intermingled with lymphocytes, plasma cells, macrophages and foreign body giant cells. (H&E, ×40)

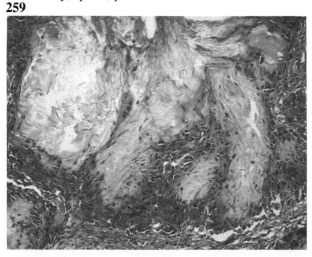

260 Chronic gouty arthritis of the hands. Note the extensive destruction of bone by urate deposits and the large soft tissue tophi.

260

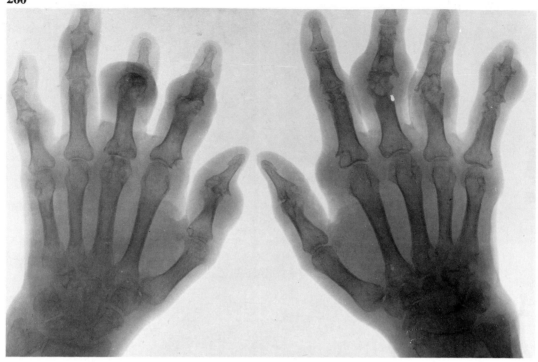

261 Urea cystals in gout. Taken with yellow parallel to the compensator and blue at 90° to the compensator.

261

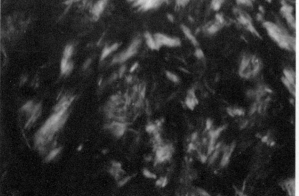

262 Chondrocalcinosis. Calcium pyrophosphate crystals to be distinguished from urate crystals in gout, with weak positive birefringence, taken with blue parallel to the compensator.

262

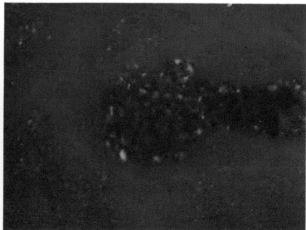

Coeliac disease

This relatively common cause of growth failure and fat malabsorption in childhood and adult life is due to enzyme deficiency or immunologic response in which there is a sensitivity to gluten, a water-insoluble fraction in wheat, barley, rye, buckwheat and malt. Exclusion of these items from the diet results in cure. Attractive and nutritionally adequate dietaries are available.

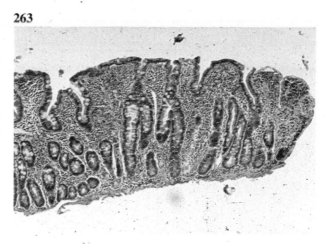

263

263 Coeliac disease. The jejunal biopsy of this adult case shows virtual absence of villi, long hyperplastic crypts of Lieberkuhn, abnormal cuboidal epithelial cells with an excess of lymphoid cells in the lamina propria; predominantly plasma cells, but lymphocytes, macrophages, eosinophils and mast cells are also present. (H&E, ×25)

Part 5   Food Toxin Disorders

There is a very large group of disorders resulting from the consumption of food that contains a toxin. This may be due to a toxin that is produced by the foodstuff; sometimes remaining in the food as a result of inadequate processing. Other disorders occur because of the contamination of food by a toxin, either due to improper storage or during processing. A further group are caused as side effects of substances that are deliberately added (food additives) to food during processing with some beneficial effect in mind, such as improving keeping quality, analeptic properties, prevention of growth of pathogens, or facilitation of processing.

The disorders presented here are illustrative of the kind of problems that arise and do not constitute an exhaustive account of this vast subject.

Chronic alcoholism

Prolonged excessive consumption of ethanol may lead to damage of most tissues in the body. Secondary nutritional deficiencies are common, especially of thiamin (**80**) and niacin (**84**). One gram of ethanol provides 7 kcal of energy and alcoholic subjects tend to be obese (**227**). Cobalt toxicity has been reported in beer drinkers (**220**).

264 Alcoholic fatty liver. The liver is enlarged, smooth, yellowish in colour and obviously fatty. The hepatocytes around the central vein become filled with small vacuoles of triglyceride and appear paler than the surrounding hepatic parenchyma. Inflammatory cells surround the area of fatty deposition. The weight of evidence suggests that ethanol is a direct hepatotoxin, although in many patients chronic nutritional deficiency probably contributes.

264

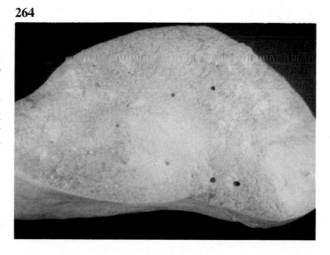

265 Fatty infiltration of the liver. In this section from an alcoholic patient the fat is stained by Sudan red.

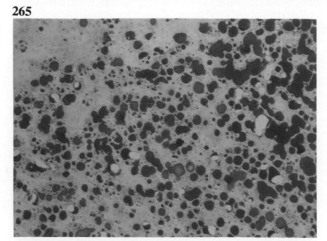

265

266 Alcoholic micronodular cirrhosis. This is the form of cirrhosis most characteristic of alcoholism. As the lesion evolves the liver decreases in size and becomes progressively nodular to produce a 'hob nail' pattern. It is yellow-orange in colour and diffusely scarred, beginning about the portal areas and eventually extending to interconnect adjacent portal triads.

267 Fetal alcohol syndrome. Abnormality of the palpebral fissures, shown here, is characteristic of this syndrome first described in 1973 in the off-spring of chronic alcoholic mothers.

   In addition cranio-facial, limb and cardio-vascular defects have been reported and there is prenatal-onset growth deficiency and develop-mental delay.

266

268 Fetal alcohol syndrome. 3 years 9 months child also with strabismus and asymmetric ptosis.

267

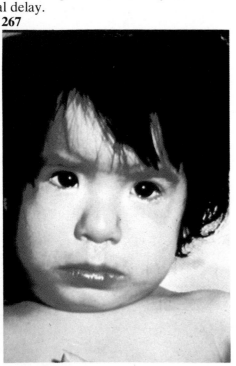

268

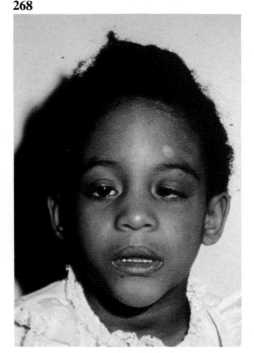

269   Fetal alcohol syndrome. This six months old female shows several characteristic signs; hypertelorism, strabismus, small nose, long upper lip with narrow vermilion border.

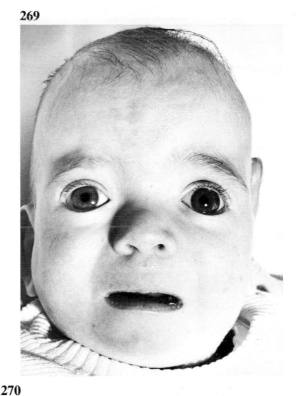

Akee fruit (Blighia sapida)

270   Consumption of akee nut produces a severe, often fatal, form of hypoglycaemia. Although the fruit is widely distributed in the tropics, most cases have been reported from the Caribbean where the disease is known as Jamaican vomiting sickness. The toxic compound is a breakdown product of hypoglycin in the nut. It blocks the access of long chain fatty acids to carnitine, necessary to their transport into mitochondria for oxidation. It also blocks the participation of pyruvate in gluconeogenesis. As these two sources of energy are blocked glycogen stores are rapidly depleted, and severe hypoglycaemia ensues.

270

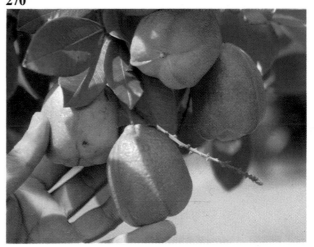

Ergotism

271 The fungus *Claviceps purpurea* commonly infects rye, as shown here, and less often wheat, barley and oats. Two distinct forms of ergotism occur, the gangrenous and convulsive, depending upon the combination of active *laevo* ergotamine compounds.

Vast epidemics of 'Saint Anthony's fire' from consuming contaminated crops in time of food shortage occurred in the past, and small outbreaks continue to be reported.

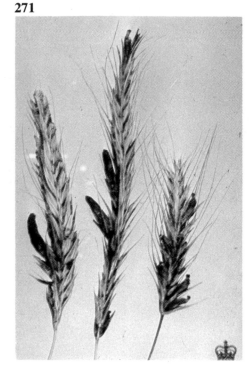

271

Glycoside toxicity

272 Cyanogenic glycosides occur in various plant tissues including cassava tubers from which they are usually leached out by prolonged soaking. Failure to do this is considered to be responsible for a syndrome consisting of ataxic polyneuropathy, amblyopia and tinnitus occurring in parts of Nigeria and other cassava-consuming regions. Highly toxic alkaloidal glycosides called solanines are produced by greening and sprouting potato tubers, consumption of which may be responsible for many mild episodes of gastro-enteritis, and coma and convulsions have occasionally been reported.

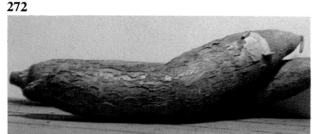

272

Aflatoxicosis

273 Aflatoxins are produced by the fungus *Aspergillus flavus*, a frequent contaminant of improperly stored groundnuts, as shown here, and some other foodstuffs. Liver cancer results from feeding contaminated groundnut to several animal species experimentally. There is some evidence for an association with hepatoma in man in parts of Africa and Asia where this is a common form of cancer.

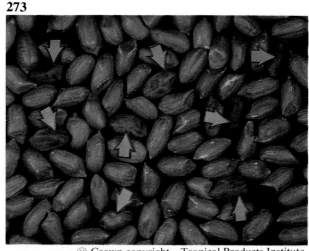

273

274 Reye's syndrome. This is a highly fatal disease of uncertain aetiology in young children, with massive fatty infiltration of the liver, as shown here, and encephalopathy. In northern Thailand epidemics of this condition have been attributed to the consumption of glutinous rice contaminated with aspergillus fungus.

274

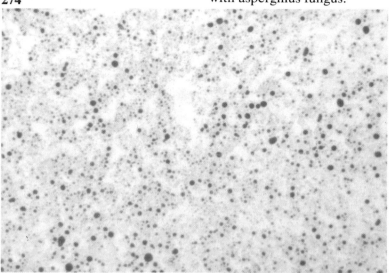

Datura poisoning

275 The tonga plant, *Datura sanginea*. Six cases were reported from Cornwall recently from eating the leaves or brewing a tea. The principle alkaloids are hyoscine, atropine and hyoscyamine. Visual hallucinations occur. Gastric lavage and sedation lead to recovery.

275

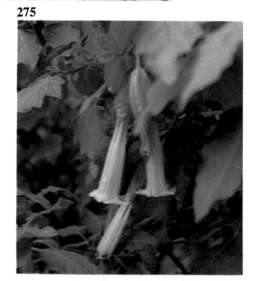

Part 6   Disorders of Uncertain Aetiology

Among the many diseases of which the aetiology is uncertain at the present time there are a number in which there is some evidence that nutrition and diet are involved in some way.

Diverticular disease

276 Diverticular disease. External appearance shows marked hypertrophy of the muscularis.

276

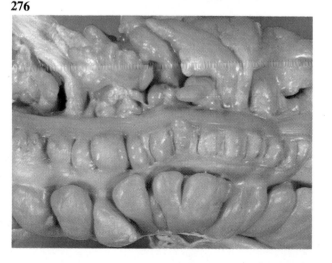

277 Diverticular disease. Viewed from the serosal surface there are numerous outpouchings aligned along one margin of the taenia coli. The sigmoid colon is most commonly and seriously affected. About 10% of all people in the West over the age of 40 are affected, rising to about 65% in old age. Many are asymptomatic. Diverticulitis causes left lower quadrant pain and repeated attacks result in fibrotic colonic narrowing.

Communities consuming a diet high in fibre content rarely have diverticular disease or other conditions associated with constipation and increased intraluminal colonic tension, such as haemorrhoids, varicose veins, pelvic vein thrombosis and appendicitis. Wholemeal bread and vegetables are good sources of fibre.

278 Diverticular disease. X-ray appearance of the most commonly affected sigmoid colon showing barium-filled diverticulae.

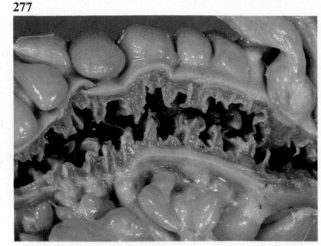

277

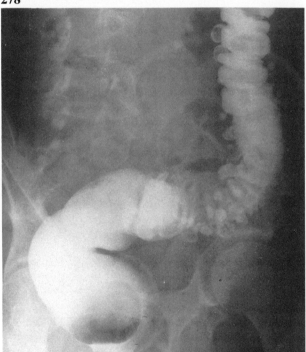

278

Endomyocardial fibrosis

279 Endomyocardial fibrosis. This is a common cause of heart disease in parts of Africa and elsewhere in the tropics. The cause is unknown but nutritional factors have been suspected as patients are usually malnourished. The process affects the endocardium of the apices of the ventricles, extending into the cusps of the atrioventricular valves as shown here. It presents in three clinical forms; mainly left sided as mitral incompetence; right sided with features suggestive of constrictive pericarditis, and involving both sides of the heart presenting as congestive heart failure.

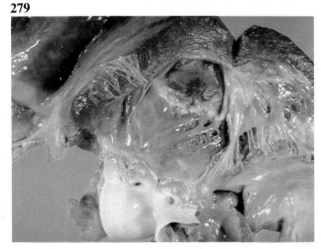

279

Cancrum oris (Noma, infective gangrene of the mouth)

280 Undernourished subjects, especially young children, tend to show unusual patterns of infection such as generalized herpes simplex infection, severe reaction to measles (**10 & 56**), anergic and afebrile reactions to infection and, as in this condition, gangrene rather than suppuration. Impairment of the immune response is thought to be responsible. Vincent's organisms, *Borrelia vincenti* and fusiform bacteria are invariably present in cancrum oris. The lesion usually starts as an area of ulcerating stomatitis with a tender, firm swelling of the upper gum and underlying maxilla and some swelling of the overlying part of the face. The teeth become loose, and inflammation spreads into underlying bone with osteitis and a sequestrum. The cheek usually ulcerates, producing a cavity leading directly into the mouth. Good diet and antibiotics result in eventual healing but usually with gross disfigurement. Occasionally the process starts in the nose, vulva or elsewhere.

281 Cancrum oris. A healed case with less deformity than frequently seen.

Cystic fibrosis

There is generalized dysfunction of exocrine glands. Inheritance is autosomal recessive. Pancreatic enzyme replacement therapy is indicated but dietary support is of great importance. Energy intake should be above normal, protein also but not excessive. Fat soluble vitamins require supplementation.

282 Cystic fibrosis. The chronic malabsorption of fat usually results in severe secondary undernutrition. This section of the pancreas shows the typical appearance of dilated ducts, containing inspissated secretion, fibrosis and disappearance of acini.

280

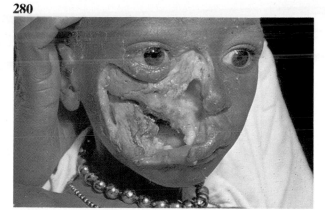

281

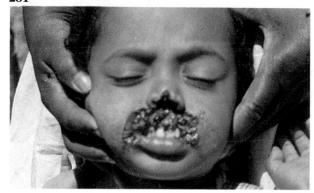

283 Cystic fibrosis. The lungs show emphysema, general and focal, thickened peribronchial markings and coarse nodular opacities throughout, denoting patchy bronchopneumonia in bronchiectatic lungs. The nutritional state usually correlates with that of the lungs rather than that of the pancreas.

283

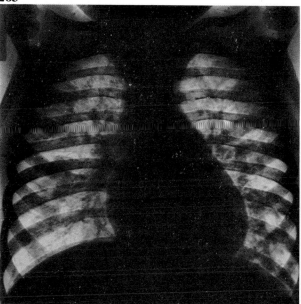

282

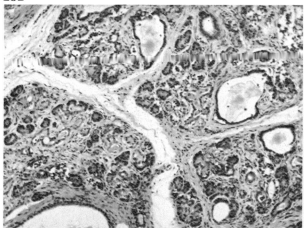

Urinary bladder stone

284 These are most commonly found in young boys and are usually composed of urates. Unlike calculus formation elsewhere in the urinary tract they occur with high frequency only in certain parts of the world, from some of which they have disappeared. At present they are common in Northern Thailand where this picture was taken, North India and parts of the Near East. Nutritional factors, especially vitamin A deficiency, have been invoked but without good evidence. There is oxalate crystaluria and this has been reduced and episodes made less frequent by increasing dietary phosphate intake. It has been suggested that phytate in a high cereal diet may chelate phosphate.

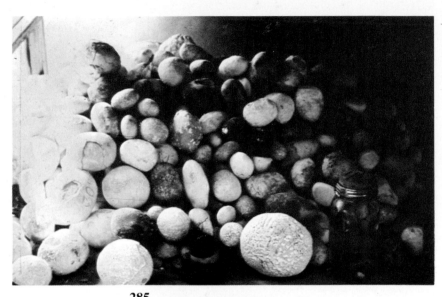

Discrete Colliquative Keratopathy (DCK)

285 This term was applied to a painless, non-inflammatory localized perforation of a small area of the cornea, frequently with a small prolapsed knuckle of iris by the writer from his experience with a number of cases in East Africa in the early 1960s. It had previously been described in South Africa as 'malnutritional keratitis' although there is no definite evidence that nutritional deficiency plays a part. Young children are usually affected. The condition spontaneously heals, unlike keratomalacia (see **61–63**) leaving a small leucoma and vitamin A is not effective. This is an active lesion.

285

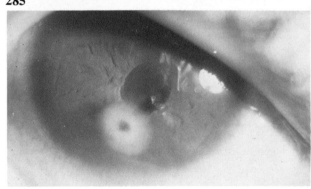

286 Discrete Colliquative Keratopathy (DCK). Typical healed lesions.

286

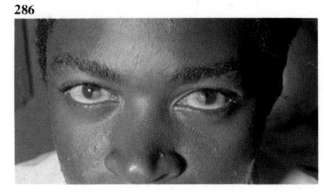

Osteoporosis

This condition is extremely common in late middle and old age. It is associated with negative calcium balance unresponsive to vitamin D therapy. A high calcium, high protein diet may lead to some improvement. Oestrogen therapy may be of benefit in post-menopausal women. Reports of increased bone density from fluoride therapy have not been generally confirmed.

287 Osteoporosis. Almost the entire skeleton is usually affected but changes are most marked in the spine and pelvis. There is loss of bone mass, with thinning of the cortical bone, reabsorption of cancellous bone spicules and enlargement of the medullary cavity. Microscopically there is no evidence of new bone formation, the bone cortex is thinned and the trabeculae are narrow and delicate.

287

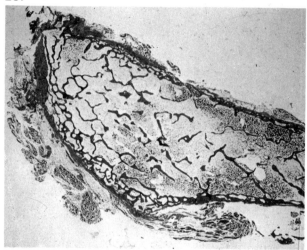

288 Osteoporosis. X-ray appearance of the lower leg with marked loss of density of the shafts of the tibia and fibula, and characteristic sharpening of the outlines of the small bones of the foot.

288

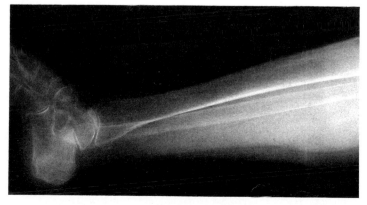

Selected bibliography

Davidson, S., Passmore, R., Brock, J.F. and Truswell, A.S. (1979). *Human Nutrition and Dietetics*. 7th edn. Churchill Livingstone, Edinburgh.

Goodhart, R.S. and Shils, M.E. (1980). *Modern Nutrition in Health and Disease*. 6th edn. Lea and Febiger, Philadelphia.

McLaren, D.S. (1981). *Nutrition and its Disorders*. 3rd edn. Churchill Livingstone, Edinburgh.

McLaren, D.S. and Burman, D. Editors. (1976). *Textbook of Paediatric Nutrition*. Churchill Livingstone, Edinburgh.

McLaren, D.S. (1980). *Nutritional Ophthalmology*, Academic Press, London.

Garrow, J.S. (1978). *Energy Balance and Obesity in Man*. 2nd edn. Elsevier/North Holland, Amsterdam.

Stanbury, J.S., Wyngaarden, J.B. and Fredrickson, D.S. Editors. (1978). *The Metabolic Basis of Inherited Disease*. 4th edn. McGraw-Hill, New York.

Addresses

The Nutritional Foundation Inc., 489 Fifth Avenue, New York, New York 10017

British Nutrition Foundation, 15 Belgrave Square, London SW1

Nutrition Society of the U.K., Chandos House, 2 Queen Anne Street, London W1M 9LE

Xerophthalmia Club, Mrs A. Pirie, Nuffield Laboratory of Ophthalmology, Oxford, U.K.

World Health Organization, Nutrition Unit, 1211 Geneva 27, Switzerland

Food and Agriculture Organization, Food Policy and Nutrition Division, Rome, Italy

American Institute of Nutrition, 9650 Rockville Pike, Bethesda, Md 20014

UNICEF, United Nations Plaza, New York, New York 10017

Swedish Nutrition Foundation, Box 641, 751 27 Uppsala, Sweden

Index

References printed in medium type are to page numbers and those in **bold** are to picture and caption numbers.